BLIND TRUST IN DOCTORS AND WHY ITS KILLING YOU

Medical Myths, lies and Misconceptions you've blindly believed about health fitness and weight loss. A patient's guide to preventative medicine and why it could save your life.

Howard Mason

Table Of Contents

Introduction

Let me set the scene for you:

You're sitting in a doctor's office awaiting your turn to go in and see him. This is the third time you've been here with the same problem. The last time you were here he prescribed you some expensive drugs and assured you that you'd feel better once you started taking them. You did everything the doctor told you to. You even got those expensive drugs, but now you're back. Why? Because you still aren't feeling better and it's all the doctors fault. He must have prescribed you the wrong medicine, right? Or maybe he was wrong about what illness you have. Or maybe it's both.

We've all been in this situation or one similar to it at some point. We trust our doctors and the people whose job it is to protect us and guard our health. Why shouldn't we trust them? After all, they get paid to make sure we're healthy.

That is the exact reason why we cannot trust them.

The medical industry and everyone involved in it makes money off of our health. If we were to become healthy, we wouldn't need them anymore and then they would stop making money. They rely on the public's illness and inability to get better on thier own. Without us they would be out of a job. So no, we cannot trust our doctor or anyone in the medical, food, or weight-loss and diet industries. There are some good doctors out there, but the majority of them are just looking out for themselves at the end of the day and we can't and shouldn't trust them with our lives.

This is one of the biggest problems we have to deal with today.

Who do we trust with our bodies, health, and lives? The only person we can fully trust is ourselves. The medical industry is just out to make money and they can't make money off of the healthy. The food industry is just a part of the medical industry and they're out for the same thing. They control what we think is okay to eat so we spend money on the things they want us to buy. The weight-loss and diet industries are no better. They create new and improved diets for people to try with little to no scientific research to back what they're saying. Only one word screams loud enough in their ears for them to hear: profit. Since everyone out there is just out to make as much profit as possible, the only person you can trust is yourself.

It's up to you to take care of your own body and your own health. This isn't just something you can do, of course. Medical professions study for years to be able to tell you what's wrong with you and they still get it wrong sometimes. What we can do is listen to what these people have to tell us but then take every single word through a strainer. Use this strainer as a way to find out the truth. Let all the lies seep through until only the absolute truth remains.

These days we have a lot of information that is readily available to us. All we have to do is type out our question and search through all the answers until enough of them match up and ring out as true. That is how we can combat the pool of lies these industries have us swimming in.

We can ask them questions, but sometimes we forget that we can. I was once like that, but one day I decided that what they were telling me wasn't good enough. I wanted to know more, so I started asking questions. Eventually I gave them questions that they couldn't even answer, so I had to go find the answers myself. I've spent years learning all that I can about the body and how it works. I've learnt all the ways we can keep our bodies healthy. I found out about all the 'facts' that the doctors were telling me and realized that they weren't facts but myths. The world of health is filled with myths. That was the hard part, but I found them all.

Once you get through all the myths and the lies, you start to see the truth. I managed to find the truth and with it I have changed my life for the better. I am healthy, fit, and this is all without the help of diet and medical companies. You can do it, too. I vow to show you through all the myths and lead you on the path to the cold, hard truth. There will be bumps and stops along the road but eventually I will help you free yourself from the money grabbing clutches of the big industries.

I can not only point out the myths and lies they use to control you. I can also show you the only truth you will ever need to know. When we're finished you'll be healthy, fit, and have a better lifestyle, one that is worth living to its fullest. This is my promise to you.

I urge you now to take the first step on your journey to the truth. The longer you wait, the more your body and mind will be poisoned. The best time to start is now. Don't put it off until you're feeling better or until you don't have anything on your plate. If you want to improve your lifestyle and become less dependent on your doctors, then this is the best place to start.

Take my hand and let's get going on this long and hard journey. Through all the mistakes, trials, and errors you will see that it is all worth it. You will be rewarded if you take action and take charge. Your life and your future belong to you and only you. Why should you not take complete control over them?

Chapter 1:
Can You Trust Your Doctor's Advice?

We all want to trust our doctors and why shouldn't we expect that we can? Doctors spend several years in medical school training and learning everything they know, but that doesn't mean they know everything. They especially don't know everything that is good for you. I would like to tell you that you can trust your doctor. In fact, in most cases you can. They do know more about what is going on inside your body and how to fix certain problems you may be suffering from. However, the problem comes in the information they have but don't want to share or the information that is out there that they don't want to acknowledge.

Your Doctor is Only Human

Humans aren't perfect, and anyone who believes differently is kidding themselves. Doctors are only human and that means that they aren't perfect either. People make mistakes, and that includes the so called 'experts' in their fields. Anyone can make a mistake. Your accountant could make a mistake, your plumber could mess up, and in the case of your doctor, when they make a mistake it can be fatal. These are the extreme cases, though.

There are plenty of stories about the doctors who have messed up or made a mistake. Some of these mistakes had huge consequences; others were minor. Still, you wouldn't want to entrust your life to someone who can easily make a mistake and put you in danger. We've all heard a story or two of how a doctor will tell their patient they're good and healthy only to see them end up in the hospital or back at the doctor's office not long afterwards.

I know a story myself of a woman who wasn't feeling very well. She went to the doctor, a man she had been trusting for years with her own and her children's lives. Her doctor said that she had the flu and it was nothing to worry about. A month later, she still wasn't well and was told she had cancer.

There's another story of a doctor who claimed one of his patient's eyes was diseased. Both the patient's eyes were perfectly fine, however the horror story comes in when the doctor goes ahead and operates on the wrong eye. There are a number of stories where doctors have made a mistake or messed up. This can be expected from any expert in their field.

Doctors have also made the opposite mistake by diagnosing their patients with a deadly disease when, in fact, one was not present. We all hope that if we do have a disease that can kill us our doctors will be able to catch it in time. Something we don't expect is for our doctors to tell us we're dying when we still have quite a lot of years ahead of us. These kinds of mistakes can lead people to live their life in fear, even after hearing that the diagnosis is incorrect, and it can cost a lot of money. Remember what I said earlier: all doctors are human, and to err is human.

Don't freak out or get scared now. Your doctor can be right and useful in some cases and you shouldn't throw their advice out altogether. What you should do is not give them any blind, unwavering faith. Take what your doctor says to you under consideration, but don't stop there. When it's your life on the line, you should always get as much involved as you can.

These days we have so much information available to us and it is more easily accessible than it has ever been. The internet is a treasure trove of information. That being said, you also shouldn't believe everything you hear or read on the Internet. There are some horror stories of people Googling their symptoms and ending up with the most extreme results. If you're going to do your research, then make sure you do it right. Remember that your doctor is only human, and so are you. Being a medical profession is hard, however that doesn't excuse the doctors from putting their patient's life in danger without knowing all the facts or while still ignoring some of the facts they do have.

After learning all of this, you can't put full blame on your doctor. They aren't the only ones in the industry. That's what the medical world has become; just another business industry.

The Business of Medicine

Earlier, I mentioned something about how someone could end up spending a lot of money when it was unnecessary. This is another problem we can find within the medical world. The world of medicine has just become another part of the business world. We can't blame the doctors for what they do. They do what anyone else does. They look out for themselves. After all, this is their livelihood and where they make the money they live on. We all want to look out for ourselves and the people we love at the end of the day. However, that doesn't excuse every action a doctor makes. They are still put in a position where people's lives are in their hands and there is a certain level of trust that needs to be held between them. The big medical pharmacies like to squeeze their way in between the doctors and their patients.

There are many medicines out there that a doctor will prescribe that are overly expensive and are used to treat the same symptoms that an even cheaper over the counter drug can treat. Medicine companies are more interested in getting you to spend your money than they are in making sure you're actually getting the medication you need. Pharmaceutical companies are million dollar businesses. It is a highly profitable industry and the people who work in the industry know this. In the end, they are no better than the stock brokers that convince you to buy high knowing very well that there is a high chance you'll lose your money.

To prove my point, we don't have to look any further than a pain medication called Vioxx. For years patients were taking this painkiller after being assured by their doctors that it would help and it was safe. After taking this medication for years to patients learned of the heart problems it causes as a side-effect. Only after suffering heart attacks because of taking the painkiller, Vioxx, did the patients start to look for who was responsible. Of course there were court cases, and punishment was handed out in the sum of some pretty hefty fines.

It was proven that the drug company that made and sold the drug knew of the effects and blatantly disregarded it and their patients. Although it is the big drug companies that should be punished, the doctors shouldn't be let off that easily. Some people found out about the heart problems that Vioxx could cause and they were not medical professionals. They learned about the effects and stopped taking the drug long before anyone else, including doctors, knew about it. What I'm trying to say is that if these doctors actually cared enough, then they would have found out about the effects. If someone who is not a medical professional can learn about the effects of a drug, then a doctor should be able to see those effects long before they prescribe the drug to their patients.

Doctors don't do that. At least, not all of them do. They like to hide behind what the big medicine companies have told them. They also place their blind faith in what they are told. We need to make sure we do not do the same.

This is not an attempt to bash doctors or medical professions and make you untrustworthy of them forever. This is just me asking you to open your eyes and see what is in front of you. You wouldn't fully trust your money with someone else. You wouldn't trust your children with someone you don't know. Don't fully trust your life and your health to a doctor.

What is Prescribed for You and What is Good for You

These two things are not always the same. The doctor may say he knows what you need to feel better and he'll prescribe you some medication that should help. However, when they are writing that prescription, they're mostly thinking about what they think is wrong with you and the money you're going to spend on the drugs. They aren't thinking about how the drug may affect you in other areas.

Maybe you're trying to lose weight and the doctor prescribes you a drug that increases your cravings and appetite. Perhaps you have bad skin and the drug you've been prescribed can make your skin even worse. This has happened to me before.

I was on a diet and on my way to losing weight when my doctor gave me some medication that increased my cravings. The medication was working for my illness but at the same time I was eating uncontrollably and gaining weight like there was no tomorrow. Not long after realizing that it was the medication that caused my cravings, I also learned that there was another drug with the same effects as the one I was taking. This drug wasn't that much cheaper than the one I was taking but it could have gotten the job done without increasing my cravings and making me gain weight. My point here is that a doctor will prescribe you the correct medication to help you with whatever problem you are having, but that doesn't mean that it's all around good for you.

It's always good to ask your doctor questions about the medication they want you to take. Up to 96% of patients in the

U.S. don't ask questions about their medication. This is an astounding number of people who are blindly taking medication because they just trust that their doctor knows what they're doing. You have a right to ask as many questions as you want. It's your body and your health on the line.

Basically, don't be afraid to ask questions. Don't just ask your doctor more about the medication he is prescribing you, ask your pharmacist as well. The truth is that the pharmacist has probably been studying drugs longer than the doctor has so ask both of them all the questions you want.

When your doctor wants you to take a medication, ask him and your pharmacist for all of the possible side-effects the medication may have. Ask them if there is another cheaper option available or an option that has fewer side-effects. Once you've asked your questions and gotten your answers, don't stop there. Do your own research. Find out everything there is to find out then cross check that information with what your doctor is telling you to see if they match.

It's usually a good idea to listen to what your doctor tells you and to follow their advice. However, that doesn't mean you have to blindly trust in them. Without even going into detail, or mentioning any horror stories, I can tell you that a doctor simply won't tell you everything. They won't tell you about the expected side-effects of a medication unless you ask them. They won't tell you about those cheaper over the counter options that will give you the same results. It's better for them if you choose the more expensive prescription drugs. Remember that your doctor is just like you and me. They're only human and they're looking out for themselves and their families. That's what we all do. Don't let this put you off doctors completely because at the end of the day we do need them. What we don't need is to put all of our trust and faith in them, as if they are perfect and won't make a mistake.

Chapter 2:
Pharmaceutical Corruption

Let's talk about the medical industry and Big Pharma. These are the people who are trusted with our health. We all trust the medical industry with our lives. but should we? We are led to believe that they are here to heal us and that they actually care about our health. This, however, is not true. We talked about doctors earlier and how we cannot trust them blindly. Even if there are some good doctors out there that actually care about their patient's well-being, those few doctors are powerless against the Big Pharmaceutical companies.

These companies own the entirety of the medical world, including everything and everyone that has anything to do with it. This wouldn't be that much of a problem if they weren't all riddled with corruption. For the pharmaceutical companies it's not about making people feel better, or about finding a cure for a disease. For them it's all about the profit. They don't care to cure a disease or heal the people because the moment someone stops needing their medicine, then they stop making money. So, let's talk about how Big Pharma are killing us instead of healing us. Let's talk about how they own and control every part of the medical industry.

Big Pharma

Although Big Pharma has a tight grip on the medical industry, they are still a new idea. The big pharmaceutical companies have been in their position of power for a short amount of time. Still, in this time they have become guilty of many unforgivable crimes, and that is including murder. The way Big Pharma is designed means that a small number of people or families are able to own all of it. I hope this sounds as ridiculous to you as it does to me. A small number of families are the shareholders of the biggest contributors to our medical industry. This small number of families is the owner of the majority of the world. That screams corruption.

John D. Rockefeller is the prime founder of the industry, a man who made the majority of his money through his Standard Oil Company. Rockefeller was quoted once saying that 'competition is a sin,' so he was responsible for removing all of the competition that the medical industry had to offer him. He used his petrochemical products to create chemicals which were later sold as medicine, and this was just the start of his mission to control and corrupt the medical world.

Rockefeller offered extremely large grants to universities so he could control the medical schools and their publications. This was just the start of the corruption. Every natural remedy or product is outlawed or patented to further their control and power over the industry. They control every medicine that is released to the public and this is the way they generate the most profit possible.

Rockefeller has already been found guilty of corruption, racketeering, and illegal business practices by the Supreme Court of the U.S. This does not stop him from channeling huge amounts of profit into the hands of the few shareholders. That's what matters to them: profits.

They call the shots and they own the world. Proof of this can be found in the lobbyist nature of the medical industry. They spend a lot of money influencing the government to make sure that the right laws are pushed forward so that their profit can be maximized. The medical industry once spent close to $240 million on lobbying. This is how much money they have to give in order to ensure that they remain in control. They spend about $56 billion dollars a year on pharmaceutical marketing in the U.S. If you think about how much money they spend on this and other ridiculous things a year, then you can see for yourself exactly how much profit they make in order to keep spending like this.

We are Clients, not Patients

With the big pharmaceutical companies running on their need for money and profit, it's not hard to see how we have ceased to be patients. We are no longer seen as the sick and the dying. We are seen as clients with pockets filled with money. It makes much more sense for them to treat a disease rather than cure it. The moment someone is cured of their disease is the moment they stop giving their money to the Big Pharma. First and foremost, the reason for the industry is to generate as much profit as possible. They can achieve this through expensive pills and procedures. This is why they suppresses natural remedies or cheaper, over the counter solutions. These natural remedies and cost effective cures make no money for the industry, which makes them useless.

We know that these natural remedies work because there are tests and studies that prove it. Not to mention that these remedies are all that were available to our ancestors who survived many diseases and illnesses. However, this knowledge is kept suppressed and hidden from the public. If we were ever to find out about these cheaper, more natural options, the medical industry would lose most of its clients and profit.

It's in Big Pharma's best interest to keep us as ignorant and dependent on them as possible. That is their goal. They keep us trusting and keep us spending our money on them. That's why when you go to the pharmacist all you will find are endless shelves filled with expensive drugs and you never just need one of them. You will always need more. The drugs are designed to treat one symptom of the disease so you are forced to buy multiple medicines to treat all of your symptoms. That is how much the medical industry has fallen.

The Control

Big Pharma is in full control of medication. They control the research, development, and creation of all medication that reaches the market. The medical industry owns almost everything. Through corruption they control the medical universities which means that most of the doctors that those universities teach belong to Big Pharma. They control the publication of medical journals and research so that anything they don't want the public to see will never get published.

A former editor of the New England Journal of Medicine said, "The medical profession is being bought by the pharmaceutical industry, not only in terms of practice of medicine, but also in terms of teaching and research."

The universities, researchers, and physicians are allowing themselves to be bought and paid for by Big Pharma. The most important journals in the medical world are also corrupt, a truth that editors slowly found out over the decades of working for them.

A big step in controlling the medical industry involves the publication of medical research, or should I say the 'selective publication.' Richard Horton, an editor of the Lancet, said, "Much of the scientific literature, perhaps half, may simply be untrue."

The medical industry controls what is published so they can control what the people believe about certain medications and drugs. The research itself is paid for by the pharmaceutical companies and they almost always have positive results. Does that not sound suspicious? Trials run by the medical industry have a 70 percent chance of their research showing a positive result. They are 70 percent more likely to have a positive result than research that is government funded. Let's think about that. The numbers just don't make sense.

Negative trials are research projects on a certain drug that show that the drug had no benefit. Negative trials are the ones being suppressed. That's why the positive trial rate is so high, because more of the positives are being published while the negatives are being swept under the rug. The evidence lies in the publication of studies for antidepressants. Of the favorable studies found, 36 out of 37 of them were published. The studies that weren't favorable to the antidepressants were not so lucky, as only 3 out of 36 were published. With these numbers, it shows that 94 percent of studies will find drugs favorable. However, in truth, only 51 percent of the studies were positive.

The company Sanofi completed 92 studies in 2008. Only 14 of them were published! That is because the people in control of what studies get published are the people who complete the studies. That's right, Sanofi were the ones that chose which of their studies were published. If a company is given that much control, what do you think they would do? They would publish the studies that benefit them the most, the studies that favor the drugs they want to sell to up their profits. They wouldn't publish something that could potentially harm them and their profits.

The main point of the fact is that Big Pharma corrupts and controls the publication of this research so they can rush their medication to the market while going through as little testing as possible. This puts everyone's life in danger. They don't care about that though. All they care about is the profit.

Along with selective publication, another way the industry is controlled is through rigging the outcomes of these trials. Before 2000, these companies were not expected to declare what end points they measured while doing their trials. End point measurements are analytic measurement at the end of a chemical reaction. This is opposed to making the measurement during the reaction. What the companies would do during their trials is they would measure as many end points as possible and simply choose the one they thought looked the best. Once they did this, they declared the trial a success. If you measure all of your research this way, then you're bound to get a positive result at some point.

In the year 2000, the government made a move to stop this from happening. They made it a requirement for companies to register what they were measuring. Before the government did this in 2000, up to 57 percent of trials had a positive result. After 2000 when the companies were forced to declare what points they were measuring, only 8 percent of the trials showed positive results. If this evidence does not further cement the belief in the corruption of the medical industry, then what will?

Murdered by Medication

It's hard to believe that something that is meant to heal us can actually end up doing more harm than good. A recent study claims that more than 250,000 people in the U.S. die every year from medical errors; however, other studies claim the numbers to be much higher, closer to 440,000 to be exact. The people in the medical industry are known to put their own needs ahead of the safety of their patients. There are many examples of this happening in the history of the medical world.

Opioid Crisis:

One of the most notable instances of this happening is with the opioid crisis. Opioids are addictive drugs that were pushed into the market, ignoring their addictive and dangerous properties, for the simple reason that they were extremely profitable. The sales of prescription opioids earned the medical industry up to

$11 billion in the U.S. annually. This nice profit helped Purdue Pharma, a big American pharmaceutical company, to overlook the fact that their drug was contributing to over 15,000 deaths by overdose.

Defective Vaccines:

Vaccines are something everybody knows about and not everybody agrees with. There are many rumors saying that they don't actually do anything to benefit us and there are also rumors saying that they can help us live better lives. The number of vaccines that are given to children has risen to extremely high levels. Children are vaccinated when they are born and we are given vaccines at intervals throughout our lives. A full lifetime's worth of vaccines can easily equal to 100. We allow this, and yet we do not trust them, and for good reason.

There are a lot of red flags surrounding the vaccines. One of the biggest is that any family in the U.S. is not legally allowed to sue any pharmaceutical company for an injury or death caused by the vaccines. These corporations cannot be legally held responsible for any harm caused by their vaccines. That is possibly one of the biggest red flags you can find.

In Australia, a child can be given up to 32 vaccines before they even reach the age of 1. Australians also have a vaccination schedule which requires them to get a vaccination at specific intervals in their life. In some places you don't have a choice on whether or not you want to be vaccinated.

Another thing strange about the vaccines is that a child is vaccinated at birth for hepatitis B. This disease is usually transmitted by sharing needles or having sex. Why are they vaccinating children for a disease that can only be transmitted through sex and sharing needles? Because it means profit. All of this adds up to a lot of profits for the Big Pharma.

The case of herd immunity is often made when discussing the importance or need of vaccines. The concept is that if the whole herd, in other words a very high proportion of the population, is immune to a certain disease, we can ensure that no one falls ill with disease and it will eventually die out. This is often used to justify the use of vaccinations. However, there are a few flaws in this concept.

In countries like the U.S. and Australia, a lot of people are flying in and out of the country on a regular basis. More often than not, a large part of the population includes tourists and yet none of them are checked for vaccinations. They could be bringing in any kind of disease which would go against the concept of herd immunity, but this concept is still used religiously by Big Pharma to justify their vaccinations. The concept of herd immunity is flawed and the vaccines are defective. The pharmaceutical companies know this and the government helps them get away with it by protecting them from legal actions.

Medical Errors:

It's not just drugs that kill people. Often, people are killed by the doctors or nurses themselves. These are medical errors. It's already been discussed that people make mistakes, but some errors cannot be excused. Many people have died in their hospital bed or during surgery because a medical professional made the smallest of mistakes. One such case was that of a little girl only 2 years old. She was diagnosed with an abdominal tumor. After various surgeries the tumor was removed and the little girl was declared cancer free. To be sure the doctors insisted that she go through her last trial of chemotherapy. Her parents eventually agreed.

It was a three-day treatment and on her final day the pharmacy technician prepared the intravenous bag. He somehow managed to fill it with 20 times the recommended amount of sodium chloride. The little girl was placed on life support a few hours after that and she was eventually declared brain dead. Three days later the parents had to say goodbye to their 2 year old daughter. She was fine. She had beaten cancer and was ready to live a full life, but one mistake ruined her chances at any kind of life.

This case is a sad one but it is not the only one out there. As mentioned above, 250,000 people die every year due to medical mistakes. Because of this, it is the third leading cause of death in the U.S. after cancer and heart disease.

FDA Recalls

The FDA, Food and Drug Administration, is responsible for protecting and ensuring the public's health and safety. They ensure that drugs and food released to the public meet the health and safety standards. When anything that is released to the public is found to be dangerous to the people, it is recalled by the FDA.

According to the FDA, a drug recall is the best way to protect the people from a harmful or defective product. A recall is usually a voluntary action taken by the company who has the defective or harmful drug. They can take this action at any time to remove the entire harmful or defective product from the market. The thing that we should worry about is the fact that drugs with the potential to harm us are actually released to the public before being called back by the FDA.

A lot of drugs are recalled by the FDA and most of them we do not even hear about. Some of them are recalled for minor issues but these issues, no matter how minor they are, can cause serious harm to the public. These drugs are taken through a large amount of testing and yet they are still released with these defects.

Pemoline:

This drug is also known as Cylert and it was on the market for a long time, from 1975 to 2010 to be exact. It was used to treat ADD and ADHD. The FDA released a warning that the drug can cause liver damage in 1999. The drug was later recalled completely.

Bromfenac:

This drug was also known as Duract, and it was only on the market for a year, from 1997 to 1998. It was an effective pain killer. However, in the year it was on the market it caused 12 severe liver damage cases, 4 deaths, and 8 liver transplants. When it was released the drug was labeled with a warning that it should only be taken for 10 days. However, patients were being given a dosage for longer than 10 days. Those that died or suffered from liver disease were the ones taking it for longer than 10 days. The FDA was quick to recall the drug.

Rofecoxib:

You will know this drug as Vioxx and it was on the market from 1999 to 2004. As you know, this drug increased the risk of heart attacks and strokes. It was responsible for up to 28,000 heart attacks in the U.S. It was reported that the drug caused 4 heart attacks per 1000 patients who took the drug. The company who manufactured the drug, Merck, recalled the drug voluntarily but not before it was given to more than 20 million people in the U.S.

Sibutramine:

This drug was also known as Meridia and it was on the market from 1997 to 2010. It was an appetite suppressant, but it also caused heart disease and increased the risk of stroke in the people who took it. It was called another Vioxx before it was recalled by the FDA.

Efalizumab:

Also known as Raptiva, this drug was on the market from 2003 to 2009. It was used to treat psoriasis. It was recalled when they found out it caused progressive multifocal leukoencephalopathy. This is a rare disease and it is extremely fatal. It causes damage and inflammation in the white matter of the brain and the central nervous system.

There are many more drugs that have been recalled by the FDA. Some are just as dangerous as these and some not as much. Even though these drugs were eventually recalled and taken off the market, they still managed to get there in the first place. How can something so dangerous and fatal as these drugs get to the public? With all the tests and trials these drugs are taken through, they should be deemed unsafe before they even get the chance to see the light of day. The sad truth is that they are not. The big companies that manufacturer these drugs let them pass through the radar because it is not the health and safety of the public that they are thinking about. The only thing they are thinking about is the money they stand to make from potential sales of the drug.

The corrupt system is growing bigger and the risk for harmful drugs to reach the public only grows. We can't trust the people in the system because they are owned by it. If you ever think that your doctor or the pharmaceutical companies can be fully trusted with your life, just remember this: you being sick keeps them rich. Why would they cure you if that were true?

Chapter 3:
Fat and Weight Loss

The weight loss and dieting industry is almost as powerful and as profitable as the medical industry. There are always new dieting trends and weight-loss schemes coming out. There are always new reasons to spend your money on another way to lose weight. The weight loss industry has its own giant companies just like the medical industry. These companies have been around since the start of the weight loss and dieting trend. They've changed ownership and grown larger ever since then. One of these companies is Weight Watchers, which has rebranded and changed the name to WW.

Today the world is a competitive one and with every company out there coming out with a new and rewarding way to lose weight, can we really trust any of them? All of these options are so customizable and personalized, as the companies will have you believe. They will have you believe in the miracle diet that can make you lose weight while still enjoying what you're eating. If it sounds suspicious to you, then you're able to see through the façade.

Weight loss and the miracle diets are all a lie and all of these companies' goals are purely profit driven.

The weight loss market is probably one of the most profitable markets out there. In the U.S. alone profits grew from $69.8 billion to $72.7 billion annually. Their profits grew at a rate of 4.1 percent in 2018. The forecast says that their profits will continue to grow by 2.6 percent annually straight through to 2023. That's just the beginning. Prescription obesity drugs, which are used to suppress appetite and help with weight loss, earn up to $655 million per year. It's earned that much for a long time with its profits never falling or rising for that matter. Weight loss surgeries are growing at a huge rate in the U.S. In 2018, it's estimated that 239,000 bariatric surgeries were performed. This earned the market $5.98 billion. The growth rate for these surgeries is estimated to be at 5 percent per year.

The weight loss and dieting market goes up and down with profits and losses, however the profits are usually huge while the losses are small. Every company involved in this industry works hard to keep up with current trends. They try to lie to you and tell you that you need to eat a certain way in order to lose weight, but in most cases this simply isn't true.

The Truth About Diets and Weight Loss

The weight loss industry would have you believe that weight loss can be gained by simply eating less and exercising more. This can be true in some cases, but not all of them. Many nutritionists believe that the answer lies in simply eating better and living healthier. There is no one perfect solution for everybody who wants to lose weight and be healthier. Everybody is different and we react differently to certain diets and exercise. That is something that most people in the weight loss industry won't tell you, because they'll lose money that way.

Here are some things that these companies won't tell you that could potentially help you live a healthier lifestyle and lose weight on your own.

1: Skip the Diet

It sounds weird at first, but diets can actually harm you more than they can help you. Most of the time people won't stay on a diet for their whole life. They'll diet until they've lost the weight they want to, then they'll stop or they'll try different diets until they can find one that works for them. This can cause a lot of problems. This kind of lifestyle leads to something called weight cycling in which someone will diet until they lose weight, drop the diet, then gain all of the weight back again. They'll start the process over and over. Diet and lose weight, drop the diet and gain weight, then go back on the diet again. Doing this long term can lead to some health issues such as chronic inflammation, high cholesterol, and blood pressure levels.

The best way to avoid this is to avoid diets. It's much more sustainable to develop a healthier lifestyle than it is to live on a diet. Work exercise and strenuous activities you enjoy into your life. Create a meal plan with healthier foods that you actually like and live off of that. Don't go on a diet for a few months to drop a little weight only to gain it again. Most diets are not sustainable, therefore the weight loss is not sustainable. What is sustainable is a healthy lifestyle.

2: Food Diaries Can Help

A food diary can help you keep track of your meals and can even help you lose weight more efficiently. What you eat is a big part of losing weight. It's very easy to eat the wrong thing. The point of the food diary is to document everything you eat throughout the day. In a couple of weeks you could see an unhealthy pattern forming and change it before it does any damage. If you notice that you always eat a snack in between breakfast and lunch, that might mean that your breakfast isn't filling enough and you need to change it. Perhaps you notice that you aren't eating any fruits or that all of your vegetables are in one meal a day and not spread out. A food diary can help you notice these things and change your habits.

You can keep a food diary the old way with an actually book and pen, or you can download an app on your phone. Any way that suits your lifestyle. Make sure to be honest with yourself and write down everything you eat or it won't work.

3: Portion Sizes Are Everything

It doesn't always matter what you're eating; it's the amount of it that matters. Giving up food doesn't help if the portion of food you're eating is too big. Even if you give up unhealthy food like soda and candy, the healthy food can still make you gain weight if you are overeating. The portion size of your food matters a lot more than what type of food you're eating.

Depending on your height, weight, and age, you burn a certain amount of calories a day even without exercising. You burn these calories by doing nothing. If you eat more calories than your body is burning and you're not exercising, then you will gain weight. If you eat fewer calories than your body is burning and you're exercising, you will lose weight. You can eat more calories than your body is burning and use exercise to get rid of the excess and more if you want. Just remember that portion size is important. Don't just watch what you eat, keep an eye on how much you eat.

4: Exercise!

As mentioned in all of the previous steps, exercise is the key ingredient to a healthy and sustainable lifestyle. Being more mindful of what and how much you eat, but it doesn't really matter if you aren't keeping active. The more active our body is, the more calories we burn, and the healthier we are. An active daily routine can lead to disease prevention and help you live a longer life.

There are many different ways you can keep yourself active. You can join a gym or yoga program. This is something that can keep you motivated because there are other people there to encourage you. Another way is to take up an active hobby that you can enjoy and work into your daily life. This can be anything from biking, to ice-skating, or even dancing. There are plenty of activities that can easily be added to your daily lifestyle that help keep you healthy and active. Give them all a try and see what works best for you. Remember, even the most effective diet is useless without exercise.

5: Allow Yourself a Cheat Meal

Although we all want to eat and live healthy, it's hard at first. It's hard to give up on all of those tasty meals we used to have. We know that this food isn't good for us, but that doesn't stop it from being delicious. It's important not to be too hard on yourself. You like eating pizza, a glass of that sugary drink is really refreshing, and nothing beats a bag of chips. There is no kidding ourselves about this.

We have to cut this kind of food out of our daily life because we know it is not good for our health. That doesn't mean you have to cut it out of your life completely. Allow yourself a chance to indulge. Have a cheat meal at least once a week. Allowing yourself to eat something unhealthy once in a while can actually help you on that weight loss journey. When we completely starve ourselves of the few things that we like, we are setting ourselves up for failure.

Allow yourself one meal a week in which you are allowed to cheat. Eat whatever you want. Have a pizza, or a burger, or even just some chips. Make sure it is only one meal. Some people give themselves an entire day to cheat. This can harm your end results, but one meal won't set you back. Treat this as a reward for being so healthy the rest of the week. As long as you don't go overboard, then you should be alright.

6: Resist the Empty Plate Urge

We all have the same urge to eat everything on our plate and leave it empty. We don't actually have to do this. If you choose not to eat everything on your plate, you could be starting a healthy habit that can help you in your efforts. This strategy could end up saving you up to 100 calories per meal. It doesn't sound like much in the grand scheme of things, but if you do it every day, then it will start to add up. It's a small gesture but it will have a big impact. All you have to do is resist the urge to eat that last piece of fruit or that last bit of meat.

8: Eat More Vegetables

Vegetables are good for you, we all know this. They are filled with fiber, they're low in calories, they're a good source of water, and they can make you feel full faster. A good habit for meals is to make sure that at least half of your plate consists of veggies. Make sure you eat the veggies first because they'll fill you up and save you from eating a lot of calories. This strategy can also help you cut down on the rest of the food which may not be unhealthy but is probably not as healthy as the vegetables.

9: Brush After Your Meal

This is another small gesture that can have a big impact. Brushing your teeth after you've finished eating can get the taste of food out of your mouth and signal to your body that you are done eating. This way you can cut down on late night snacks. We all sneak a snack every now and again. You won't want to do that after you've cleaned your teeth. Get into the habit of cleaning your teeth the moment you've finished eating and you will see the results.

10: Self-care

Most importantly, you have to put yourself before everything else. The diet may not be working for you and it may be harming your health, so drop it. You don't have to be obsessed with losing weight especially if it's hurting you along the way. You don't need a diet to lose weight, you just need to care for yourself. Ignore the scale for now and work on getting your life together so you're more active and eating healthier. Once you've got it all working out for you, then you can check how the numbers on the scale are.

It would be easy if there was just a diet that actually worked for everyone. That's what those big companies would have you believe. However, it's not true. Everybody is different. One diet might work for one person but that doesn't mean it will work for you as well. Diets are a lie fed to us by the weight loss and diet industry. Diets don't work when it comes to a healthy life and weight loss. Having healthy habits and living an active lifestyle is the only way to lose weight and keep it off. We may have to change our lives in order to make them healthier and sustainable but in the end, we are rewarded more for it.

Lies About Weight Loss

We've all been told a thing or two about weight loss and dieting. These things are 'facts' or things we have to do if we want to lose weight. We're led to believe that if we don't follow these certain steps, then we won't lose weight no matter what. All of these things are lies. I'm going to list these ridiculous so called 'facts' so you know to avoid listening to the people who tell you to do this.

1: Fewer Calories

Some people will say that the fewer calories you consume, the better. This is not only untrue but it can also set you up for failure. The less we eat during one meal, the more likely we are to overeat during the next meal. Not only that, but we can actually cause ourselves harm because we aren't giving our bodies enough energy. Yes, it is good to eat less but if you eat too little, you are basically starving your body of the energy and nutrients it needs to get through the day. Restricting the amount of calories you eat is not good. It's better to eat healthier and less food while still giving your body what it needs instead of starving yourself for quick results.

2: Six Meals a Day

This is on the opposite side of the scale. Instead of eating fewer calories, people spread their daily calories into six small meals a day. This can be a good idea for some people, but for others it can be bad. The reason is that everyone has a different version of what a small meal is. If your six small meals a day turn into six not so small meals a day, you'll end up overeating. Also, a Canadian study has found that this method of splitting your daily calories into six meals doesn't have that much of an effect. The research said that if you eat six meals a day rather than the usual three, it can actually make you want to eat more. If you want to try out this method then I suggest you learn everything you need to know about it first so you can follow it properly.

3: No Carb! No Fat!

A healthy lifestyle is all about balance. You can't have balance if you're taking things away from your diet. It's simple, if you take one thing away you could end up eating too much of something else. Some dieting trends ask you to eliminate an entire food group like low-fat or low-carb diets. These are the worst diets. If you cut fat out of your diet you could end up eating more carbohydrates. Carbohydrates are known for stimulating insulin which is a fat storing hormone. However, if you cut carbs out of your diet you could end up feeling sluggish or become constipated.

The trick is to monitor how much of each food group you eat, but you cannot remove an entire food group altogether.

4: Skip the Meal and Have the Juice

This is a bad idea. Some advice might tell you to swap out your meals for a juice instead. This juice is supposedly healthy and better for you. However, that juice is most likely filled with sugar and it won't fill you up. You're just going to be hungry later and end up eating more calories than you should be. It's actually better that you chew your meals because, believe it or not, chewing is a form of exercise and can actually get your metabolism going. Chew your food, don't drink it.

5: A Tablespoon of Coconut Oil a Day

I'm sure you've heard it once or twice. If you eat a tablespoon of coconut oil a day it can help you lose weight. Some people think this is a miracle cure for weight loss, but it's not. Coconut oil is saturated fat. It's basically like lard. Do you really want to eat a tablespoon of lard every day? One tablespoon of coconut oil equals 12 grams of saturated fat and 117 calories. The American Heart Association suggests that we limit our daily intake of saturated fat to 13 grams a day. One tablespoon of coconut oil is basically the entire recommended limit of saturated fat a day. If you have more you are putting yourself at risk of a heart attack.

Skip the tablespoon a day and just use it in your cooking. You'll probably end up eating a lot less of it.

6: Eat this Every Day

Some diets will tell you that you must eat a certain food every day or even with every meal. These diets should be avoided at all costs. A diet that puts focus on a certain food can be dull and lacking in certain vitamins. A diet may tell you to have a grapefruit with every meal. For the first few days it might be okay, but you'll get bored of the taste after a while and it will stimulate your cravings for some other food. If your cravings are stimulated then there's more of a chance that you will cheat on your diet and it will all be for nothing.

7: Exercise and Diet Apps

Ignore these and keep them off of your phone. Some apps claim they can calculate how much you can eat based on how many calories you burned during exercise. Just because an app tells you that you can binge eat doesn't mean you should. It's actually impossible for an app to be able to tell how many calories you burn while exercising. People exercise at different strengths and speeds which means they burn calories at different rates. One app on your phone cannot tell you how many calories you have burned, which means it can't judge what you can eat without gaining weight. Just stick to your own diet and exercise and trust that you're eating right.

8: Have a Big Breakfast

One of the most commonly heard dieting facts is that you have to eat a big breakfast. It's true that breakfast is the most important meal of the day. It gives us the energy we need for most of the day and fuels all of our early morning activities. However, a big breakfast is not necessary for this. It is possible to have too much fuel in the morning.

Instead of eating a huge breakfast in the morning, choose a normal sized breakfast with a good amount of protein in it. Protein is the food we need to energize ourselves. Things like eggs or Greek yogurt can give us all the energy we need for the day without the possibility of overeating.

9: Supplements

There is some information out there that would have you believe you can burn fat just by taking vitamin and mineral supplements. This is false, of course. You may need these supplements to replace the vitamins and minerals you aren't getting in your diet, but they do not act as miracle weight loss drugs. If you need to take them, then by all means do so but don't think they'll magically burn fat and solve your problems.

10: Detox for Weight Loss

There are a lot of detox teas or juices out there that all of these weight loss and diet companies try to sell us. They'll tell you all sorts of things like detoxing can help you lose weight. There is no scientific evidence out there that supports this information. Our bodies naturally cleanse themselves every day. What really matters is what we put into our body. Just eat natural and let your body to its job. There's no need to waste your money on those 'natural' detox products when your body already does the job.

There it is. These are the common lies a big weight loss and diet company will try to tell you so you spend more money on them. In the grand scheme of things, the weight loss industry is no different than the Pharmaceutical industry. They don't care about you. They care about profit. You're just another client who they can try and fool into spending money on countless diets that won't work. The need for a diet is probably one of the biggest lies they can tell. Diets aren't sustainable. A healthy, active lifestyle is sustainable and more affordable. Don't become a slave to the dieting industry and the scale.

The true information is out there for you to see. It is the same situation with your doctor. You don't trust him completely with your health, so you shouldn't trust these weight loss companies with your health either. Take it into your own hands.

Chapter 4:
Foods Your Body Needs and the Pyramid of Lies

The very first food pyramid was created in 1988 and it was seen as an important guideline to eating and living healthy. These dietary guidelines were written in great haste and virtually no trials nor tests were run to support them. When the first food pyramid was created there was no scientific evidence to support it. The public was spoon fed the belief that the food pyramid is the best guideline to live by. They stated that if you only ate what and how the pyramid told you to, then you would live a healthy life. However, given the fact that there was no evidence to support their claims, we can safely assume that the pyramid of food was a lie.

The pyramid of food is a visual guide used to show people what food is bad for them and what food is good for them. It takes the shape of a pyramid with the good food groups being at the base and the bad food groups occupying the top. The first food pyramid encouraged people to consume more carbohydrates and to avoid fat. These guidelines were, of course, successful. It decreased America's consumption of fat by 15 percent. This sounds like a huge success. However, with the consumption of fat reduced, why did the obesity and diabetes rates increase? The food pyramid and these dietary guidelines were meant to increase the overall health of the population. If that's the case, why is it continuing on a downward spiral with more and more Americans becoming obese and diabetic? The answer is simple; because the food pyramid is part of the big industries that rule the world.

Big Pharma, the weight loss and dietary industry, and the food industry are all part of one big machine. The food pyramid is just part of their lies to control how much the public spends and how much profit they make. Evidence for this is there for those who are looking for it.

Every five years the Dietary Guidelines must be reviewed by a panel of experts as required by the legislation. The panel must consist of 15 different experts in obesity, cardiovascular disease, nutrition, pediatrics, and public health. This panel of experts, however, cannot be trusted, and neither can their review of the Dietary Guidelines. This is because the process of selecting the panel of experts is heavily influenced by lobbying. Yes, the same lobbying we see in the medical industry happens here as well. This is evidence that the dietary system cannot be trusted. Big companies like the American Meat Institute, the Wheat Foods Council, the Soft Drink Association, and the Salt Institute are the companies behind the lobbying. These and other companies work hard and spend big to ensure that the Dietary Guidelines appear in their favor. The only reason they would invest money into something like this is if they can stand to gain more money from it. With the right influence, these companies can control what the public deems healthy. Through that, they can control what the public chooses to buy. All valid reasons to assume the Dietary Guidelines and the food pyramid are lies.

Up until recently, it was considered business and social suicide to even consider that the Dietary Guidelines may not be trustworthy. Researching it or suggesting an alternative to the system was considered crazy. Now there are some people who are willing to break down the lies and expose the Dietary Guidelines for what they are. One important contributor to this new movement is Walter Willett. He is the chairman of the Department of Nutrition at the Harvard School of Public

Health. Walter Willett is the spokesperson of a long-running diet and health study. These studies are extremely comprehensive. The studies have cost more than $100 million and have included 300,000 individual civilians. According to Walter Willet, all of the data from these studies contradicts the current "low-fat is good for your health" beliefs.

There are good fats and there are also bad fats, but the current food pyramid would have you believe that all fats are bad. They have been focused on making sure the public cuts fat out of their diet. However, most scientific evidence available to us has proven that has only caused more problems for the public's health. Walter Willett believes the lie that all fat is bad for you has contributed to America's rising rates of obesity.

The people who are willing to perform studies like this are helping the public to combat the rule these big companies have over us. It's sometimes hard to believe just how deep the corruption goes. All of these companies are run by politics and profits. They don't care about the public. We're all just customers with money. One fact that can show how shady the business world is involves the Heart Association. The Heart Association is a non-profit organization in the United States. They fund cardiovascular medical research and they try to educate the public on proper cardio care in order to reduce the risk of cardiovascular disease and stroke. The Heart Association was also founded by a company that makes and sells alternatives to butter. Those sets of circumstances are suspicious. They warn the people of the risk that the fat in butter poses for your heart and then they make money selling you alternatives to butter. This is another reason why no product or information that comes out of these big companies can be trusted.

The main point is that the food pyramid and the Dietary Guidelines have done far more bad than they have good.

America has the highest obesity rate in the world and the diabetes rate has only gotten worse. There were about 30 million diabetics in the year 1985, and now it's predicted that there is going to be 438 million diabetics in 2030 and a lot more pre-diabetics. This is all because of the misguided food pyramid.

What You Should Be Eating

We've spoken about a low-carb diet earlier. Although you shouldn't completely eliminate a food group from your diet, you can minimize your consumption of certain foods. The low-carb diet is by no means a new discovery. It's been around for over a century, but it has recently gained some traction. The low-carb diet is a good choice for combating obesity and diabetes. There are foods that diabetics shouldn't consume under any circumstances and then there are foods that are okay for diabetics to eat. Some of these foods go against the guidelines set by the food pyramid.

Butter, cheese, fish, all meat, olive oil, and all organs are foods that diabetics can eat freely. Bread, oats, flour, rice, sugar, starches, and juice are all foods that should be removed from a diabetic's diet. The foods that should be removed from a diabetic's diet actually form the base of the food pyramid. That means these are the foods you can eat freely according to the Dietary Guidelines. Vice versa, the foods that a diabetic can eat freely are restricted according to the food pyramid.

There's no problem with having fat in your diet. There are healthy fats that are actually good for you. The best way to add fat into your diet is after you've lowered your carb intake. So increase your healthy fat intake after lowering your carb intake. It's that simple. The current American diet consists of high fat and high carb which is the main cause of the obesity and diabetes epidemic. If you increase your fat but keep eating the same amount of carbs, you'll also end up on the standard American diet. So this step is probably the most important one.

It sounds weird when you hear that you should actually be eating more fat. It's not just any fat you're eating. There are good fats which provide good nutrients for your body as well as bad fats that harm your body when you consume too much of it. However, the same thing can be said of carbohydrates. There are good and bad carbohydrates but the problem is that too much of both can be harmful. The reason you shouldn't remove fat from your diet is because when you do you're removing nutrients your body needs and most of the time you're replacing the fat with something far more harmful.

When fat is removed from a food, something replaces it. Sometimes whatever is used to replace the fat is worse than the fat itself. Take cream cheese, for example. Low-fat cream cheese consists of 15 percent carbs, while regular cream cheese only has 4 percent carbs in it. Reading the label on certain foods might increase the time it takes you to shop, but you can see for yourself exactly what you're buying that way.

The fear of fat is the cause of the Dietary Guidelines we've been blindly following for nearly two generations. However, these guidelines have no scientific evidence to back them. For these two generations we've been told that reducing our fat intake, especially saturated fats, will decrease our risk of cardiovascular disease and reduce our cholesterol. Yes, saturated fat does reduce the cholesterol in our bodies but it mainly reduces the good cholesterol. Yes you heard that right. There is such a thing as good cholesterol and we need it in our bodies.

Reducing your consumption of saturated fats reduces HDL in your body which is the good cholesterol. Reducing saturated fats also makes LDL which is the bad cholesterol. Low-density lipoprotein, or LDL, is the majority of cholesterol we have circling in our bloodstream. Scientists proposed that there was a link between the LDL and heart disease. This link is the reason the Dietary Guidelines have insisted on the public lowering their fat intake. However, further studies have shown that you can reduce the amount of LDL in your body by reducing your fat intake, but this did not decrease the number of heart disease cases or mortality rates.

In short; LDL, which is bad, carries cholesterol from the liver to the body and the organs. HDL, which is good, carries the cholesterol from the body back to the liver for disposal. There have been some new studies done on reducing the LDL by having a high-fat diet and a low-fat diet. In these studies the high-fat diet was better at reducing the incidence of heart disease.

My advice would be to not ignore the food pyramid entirely, as some of its information is correct. However, not all of it can be trusted. Take all of its advice with a grain of salt. Make sure you do your homework and find out what's best for you to eat rather than trust that someone else cares enough to give you the right information. The best diet by far is the low-carb and high-fat diet.

Here are some simple tips and habits that can change the way you eat and better your lifestyle:

- When you think you're hungry take a moment to ask yourself, "Am I really hungry or am I just bored?" Learn the difference between hunger and boredom. This can lead to a lot of snacking.

- Try eating a wide variety of foods. If your meals get dull or plain, then you might end up overeating something more enjoyable. Your meals can get boring if you eat the same things all the time. Make sure your meals are healthy but try to experiment with new tastes.

- Fill your plate with non-starchy vegetables. The right vegetables are filled with fiber and they can help you lose weight and stay active. Make sure at least half of your plate is filled with non-starchy vegetables. Eat as many vegetables as possible to make sure it doesn't get bland or dull.

- Introduce a wide range of low-sugar fruits to your diet. These can make great midday snacks if you find you are feeling a little hungry in between meals.

- Make bigger dinners at night so you can save some for lunch the next day. If you make twice the amount of food you can have a good healthy dinner and then a good healthy lunch the next day. This saves time and it saves you having to decide what to have the next day. Obviously you shouldn't do this every night, as your meals could end up getting boring.

- Remember to eat healthy fats such as olive oil, butter, and avocados.

Chapter 5:
The Cardio Myth: Exercise Smart

There are a lot of myths and lies surrounding exercise. Everyone always has the 'right way' to exercise. The magazines, TV shows, and YouTube videos, are all lying. Everybody wants to be the one that knows what you can do to lose weight, but most of the knowledge out there is just a myth.

It's time that you knew the truth. There are some big lies out there, but the thing is that they seem legit enough that we automatically believe them. The logic is there, but it's still wrong. Just because it sounds right doesn't mean you should believe it. I'm going to shed some light on the biggest exercise myths so you know what to believe and what you shouldn't believe.

The Big Lies

1: Cardio Burns Fat

This is probably one of the biggest lies. You've probably heard it before. Cardio exercise is the best exercise for burning fat. It sounds like it makes a lot of sense. It gets your heart going, it makes you sweat, and it burns a lot of calories. However, it's not the best exercise for burning fat or losing weight. The thing with cardiovascular training, things like jogging, skipping, cycling, or running, is that your body can quickly adapt to it. This kind of training seems hard at first but it only takes a short while before your body adapts to the exercise. This means that you'll be burning fewer calories every time you exercise. In order to keep up and keep burning fat at a high rate, you have to increase the intensity of your cardio training more and more

43

every time you exercise. This can be dangerous and is less effective over time.

Another bad thing about cardio training is that as soon as you stop, so does the fat burning. You're only burning calories during the exercise. Other forms of training, such as weight training, still burns calories long after you've stopped exercising. To sum it up, cardiovascular training is a good form of exercise and it's a great way to stay active, but it is by no means the best exercise for burning fat. There are a lot more effective ways to burn calories and fat than cardio.

2: Walking Isn't Exercise

Of course walking is exercise! Any time your body moves you are exercising. Walking was the only form of exercise our ancestors got. Before we all were on diet trends and gym memberships we were walking. It's a great form of exercise. It falls into the cardio category but it's still exercise. Some people out there will have you believe that walking isn't proper exercise and that you need to jog and run everywhere, but they're wrong. We should all walk every day. A walk a day can keep the doctor away. Seriously though, walking is good for mental health, cardiovascular health, calorie burning, fat loss, overall well-being, and it is a sustainable activity. That's more than you can say for a lot of forms of exercise.

3: You Have to Exercise Every Day

No you don't. Whoever said that is obviously lying. This statement also depends on what you consider to be exercise. As I said earlier, any time when your body is moving and being active can be considered exercise. With that logic, we're already exercising every day. It is good to stay active. You can be active every day and exercise every day, but that could take the form of many things like walking your dog.

You don't have to go to the gym or do a full exercise routine every day. It's actually better for weight loss if you allow your body some rest time. What happens when you exercise is you're actually tearing and stretching your muscles. That's why you feel strain while you exercise and that's why you're sore the next day. This is good. What this allows your body to do is repair itself. While your body is repairing itself, it's burning more calories and fat. However, in order for your body to repair itself you have to give it the chance. That means resting for a day or so.

By all means, be active every day. Take the stairs instead of the elevator, be bubbly and move around a lot. Even if you're standing in line at the grocery store or in front of the stove in the kitchen, you can be more active. Dance a little, sway your body from side to side. Anything that gets your body moving gets your metabolism going and helps you lose weight. You don't have to go to the gym every day to exercise every day. Your body needs that rest in order to repair itself. Once it's repaired, you can go back to your normal exercise routine, but remember not to put too much of a gap in between your workouts. There is such a thing as too much rest.

4: More Pain, More Gain

This information is not only wrong, it is also dangerous. It's very easy for someone to be misled by this saying. You should never work out until you hurt yourself. There is a difference between straining yourself and hurting yourself. If you exhaust your body or train too hard you could end up seriously hurting yourself. You need to know your limits and stay under them. You will gain without pain.

That being said, you also need to know that feeling a little strained doesn't mean you should stop because you're in pain. It's important to know the difference. You will feel strain while exercising, but you can't stop the moment you feel the strain.

This part can be difficult, but once you find your limit you'll know when you have to stop and when you can keep going.

5: If It's Fun, Then It's Not Working

Who thought up this? It sounds like it makes sense, right? Exercise is sweaty and it's hard work. It shouldn't be fun. If it's fun for you then you aren't doing it right.

That's completely wrong. Exercising doesn't have to be a chore. You don't have to dread the moment you need to exercise. There are forms of exercise that you can find enjoyable and it's actually better if you enjoy it when you exercise.

Certain activities and hobbies are enjoyable and they do fall into the category of exercise. Things like biking and rollerblading are exercise and they could be enjoyable activities. The more you enjoy exercising, the more likely you'll keep at it for years. The lie everyone keeps telling about how exercise needs to be strenuous and you can't enjoy it is probably one of the most harmful lies out there.

You can enjoy your exercise and it's actually better if you do. So have as much fun with it as you can!

6: Weight Training isn't for Women

Some people would have you believe that women shouldn't do weight training. This is a silly lie. Why shouldn't women do weights? Some people might believe that weight training is meant for men, but we can argue that women can gain more from weight training than men. Weight training can help women increase their bone density, help with their mental well-being, fat loss, and body composition. One of the best advantages women can gain from weight training is the offsetting of osteoporosis.

An understandable fear that most women have with weight training is that they'll gain muscle. Not all women actually want to bulk up like men, but you don't have to worry because this won't happen easily. Women don't have the level of testosterone that men do, so they simply won't be able to gain muscle that easily. At least, not like men do, anyway. There are a lot of good things women can gain from weight training, so silly rumors like this shouldn't stop them from doing it.

7: You Have to Work Out in a Gym

I don't know who thought up this lie, but I hope it sounds as stupid to you as it does to me. Of course you don't have to work out in a gym if you want to get fit or lose weight. Our ancestors never had a gym to work out in and they did fine on their own. Nature has a gym of its own. The world around you can be your gym if you know how to use it. There are hiking, biking, and running trails, and each one can work out your body in different ways. There are also plenty of sports and hobbies out there that don't require a gym membership, things like swimming and rock climbing. So, to answer, no you don't need to work out at a gym if you want to lose weight or get fit.

8: Yoga isn't an Actual Workout

Yoga can be a pretty relaxing activity. It's supposed to be great for your mental and emotional health, but there are plenty of other benefits beyond relaxing and chilling out. Yoga is strenuous if you haven't done it before. It's a great workout with many benefits. Yoga has been known to correct posture imbalance and strengthen skeletal tissue. It can also encourage better breathing habits as well as act as an offset to injury. Yoga has even been connected to improving blood flow and heart health. Yoga is indeed great for relaxing but it's also a very beneficial workout.

9: Weight Training Can Help You Get Big

It's actually a lot more complicated than that if you want to gain muscles. Weight training does help, but there's more to it than that. You have to build your whole lifestyle around it if you want to gain some proper muscles. It takes a lot of effort. You need to eat the right food, plan the right workout, and be dedicated if you actually want to bulk up in the right way. It takes far more than just lifting weights a few times a week or when you have time. It's a whole lifestyle.

10: Lose Weight First, Then Exercise

This is probably one of the biggest and worse lies out there. It's kind of a silly one as well. Why would anyone think that you have to lose weight before you can start exercising? The main reason anyone would exercise is because they want to lose weight. Sometimes this lie is told to people who are well above the weight they should be or people who are obese. They're told that they can't start exercising until they've lost a bit of weight first. Then they're put on a diet to lose that weight but as mentioned before, diets don't work and they especially don't work if you're not exercising as well.

You don't need to lose weight before you can start exercising. Yes, you won't be able to do anything extreme until you've lost a little weight, but there are a lot of exercises out there suitable even for people who have never exercised before. As mentioned above, any time your body is active you are exercising. Don't listen to those people who say you need to diet and lose weight before you can exercise. Just start exercising. Do it today, right now. Don't let anyone stop you. The sooner you start, the sooner you can reach your goals.

The Biggest Lies

The lies above, although harmful to the world of exercising and fitness, are only small white lies. There are far more harmful myths out there. These big lies can make someone's life harder if they're trying to lose weight or get fit. They can even discourage someone and stop them from reaching their goals. Now we're going to expose these lies for what they are.

1: Calories are Calories

Calories are all anyone ever talks about when it comes to eating healthy. One of the most harmful beliefs is that all calories are the same, so you don't have to worry about what calories you eat, only how many of them you eat. Everyone is sold on the idea that they can eat what they want as long as they stay under their set calorie limit. This limit is predetermined based on their age, weight, and height. People have been made to believe that they just need to stay under the limit and then they can eat what they want. This is an extremely harmful myth.

The truth is that not all calories are the same. Some calories are more harmful than others. It's the same as having good fats and bad fats. There are good calories and bad calories, and yes it matters which ones we eat. The calories we consume give our bodies different hormonal effects. For instance, the calories you get from an M&M will give you a different hormonal effect than the calories you get from an avocado. These hormonal effects are why simply counting calories is not good enough for any kind of end result.

Your body needs fat, protein, and carbohydrates to remain in hormonal balance. There are good and bad versions of all these food groups, and you need to find a proper balance between all of them. Each one of them has a different effect on your body. Fat slows down your digestion and it increases your satiety. Carbohydrates make your blood sugar rise. Protein helps your body store body fat which is used to provide energy. We need each of these food groups for our bodies to run the way they're supposed to.

When we eat carbohydrates, our blood sugar is raised but this provides us with energy to use. The energy provided by these carbohydrates is usually used immediately, with sugar being used first. However, if you eat too much of this food group then the remaining sugar in your body that can't be used for energy is stored as body fat. This storage is controlled by the hormone insulin.

When we eat protein, all of that body fat which was stored by the insulin is then used for energy. This is done by the hormone glucagon. This hormone acts as a counter to insulin so that we don't end up with too much stored body fat. Without protein, our bodies wouldn't be able to mobilize the stored body fat into energy.

Eating fat basically helps us to feel full. It slows down our digestion and increases our satiety. Fat also slows down the rise of your blood sugar which in turn slows down the release of insulin. Eating fat can help you to limit the amount of fat that your body stores while making your body think it is full so you stop eating.

As you can see, all of these food groups help your body stay healthy and balanced. All of the things these food groups accomplish have nothing to do with the amount of calories you eat and everything to do with balancing the hormones in your body. This should be more than enough evidence to prove to you that overeating calories is not the cause of fat gain or an unhealthy lifestyle. The only cause is not giving your body the right balance of the three food groups it needs.

2: The Scale Determines Your Health

This isn't exactly a complete lie or myth, but it's not a whole truth either. People believe that the weight you see on the scale determines how healthy you are overall. While this is true with some extreme cases such as obesity, it simply isn't fully true with everyone else.

We end up spending half our time looking at the scale and feeling discouraged and unhappy with the result we see. We eat healthy and work out every day but the number on the scale doesn't always change. Sometimes the scale won't show you results even when they are there. When we exercise to get fit or lose weight, it doesn't always show on the scale straight away. The best way to avoid unnecessary disappointment is to ignore the numbers on the scale and focus on your body's composition. Your body composition is the measure of how much of your body is muscle tissue, how much of it is fat, and how much of it is water. Then there's even how much of it is bone.

What we need to do is look at our body composition. Instead of working on lowering the number on the scale, we need to work on lowering the proportion of stored fat in your body to muscle. It often happens, especially with women, when they've followed their diet precisely and they work out every day but then they step on the scale and find that they haven't lost any weight or that they've even gained weight. This can be discouraging if you don't know what's really happening. You see, muscle weighs more than fat. When you're cutting away at the fat in your body, then that fat is usually replaced with muscle. Seeing the number on the scale go up or stay where it is can lead you to believe that what you're doing isn't working and you're making no progress when that simply isn't true.

It's better to focus on how you look in the mirror rather than what the number on the scale is. You'll decrease in clothing size, but the scale may stay the same. Ignore the scale and focus on your body's composition if you want to see true results.

3: A Comfortable Workout Works

There is no such thing as a comfortable work-out. You can't stay in your comfort zone and expect to give your body what it needs to lose weight and get fit. There is a whole industry of fitness and health built around this one myth. There is no way you can achieve results without pushing yourself beyond your comfort zone.

This lie takes many forms. You can casually walk every day and lose weight. You can have abs in eight minutes. Do this 3 minute workout once a day and you'll lose weight. All you need to lose weight are shake weights. All of these and more are lies. If you want to achieve proper results it is far more difficult than that.

Every single time you put your body through a workout, it will learn and adapt to it. This means that the next time you do the same workout your body will react differently and even do it easier. This will yield few to no results over time. Once your body adapts to a certain workout, the only way to counter it is to intensify your next workout.

Every time you go for a run, you have to run faster and further. Every time you lift weights you have to increase the weight or the number of times you lift them. Whenever you do any kind of exercise, the next time you have to increase the intensity in some way. This is the only way you can counter your body's ability to adapt.

When we exercise we are asking our body to adapt to what we're doing. Basically, if you run 5 miles a day in 20 minutes, then that is what you're asking your body to adapt to. You're asking your body to change itself so you can consistently run 5 miles a day in 20 minutes. Your body's fat and muscle and your fitness level will change to match this goal only. It will never change if you don't change the intensity. Your body will reach this adaption after some repetition but once it does, there will be no further change or gain.

Therefore, a comfortable workout will never help you reach your goals. You have to push yourself. Every time your body adapts to a certain workout, you have to intensify it somehow. Don't worry though, you only have to do this until you reach your goal. Once your body has managed to adapt to the fat and muscle percentage that you want, then all you need to do is maintain that level. You won't have to intensify your workout anymore but you can't allow yourself to relax too much either. In order to maintain your body's adaptation you have to push it to the point you've reached every time you work out. If you allow yourself to get lazy or slack off, then you will only see yourself moving backwards.

Now that you know all of the lies the world of exercise and fitness have been spreading, you can keep your sights on the few truths there are. There are a few things you can do to improve your health and lifestyle. You don't need to listen to the lies people tell you even if they appear to be an expert in their field. Remember that they have something to gain from you believing what they tell you even if what they're telling you is a lie.

The only truths you need to know are these few I have told you. If anyone tries to tell you otherwise, then be very wary of them. Most often you'll find that they just have something to sell to you.

Chapter 6:
The Cholesterol Myth

We've touched on cholesterol earlier in this book. I'd like to talk about it a little more. There is a big myth surrounding the word and it can be very harmful if you don't know the full truth behind it. Cholesterol has become a bad word lately. It's understandable considering the connections it has to heart disease, strokes, and heart attacks. There is a definite connection between the two, that part is not the myth, but there is so much more to the story that isn't being told. What I told you earlier will appear again here, but I will be expanding on the science of it and the exact differences between good cholesterol and bad cholesterol. I'll also explain properly why we need cholesterol in our bodies so we can work past this myth once and for all.

In order for us to live healthy and happy lives, our bodies need to be in perfect balance. We can't eliminate cholesterol from our bodies entirely and expect to be in balance. The truth is that we need cholesterol, and more harm than good will come from eliminating it completely. The cholesterol levels in our bodies are usually used as an indication of our heart's health. However, the relationship between our cholesterol levels and the health of our heart is not set in stone. Some people who have a high cholesterol level don't seem to be affected by it at all, while others have been affected directly by their cholesterol level. This can be explained only by the fact that there are two types of cholesterol.

There are two different types of lipoproteins that our body uses to carry cholesterol from one cell to the other. One form of cholesterol is called low-density lipoprotein, or LDL, and the second form is high-density lipoprotein. The amount of both types you have in your body can be measured with a blood test, and obviously it matters how much of each one you have.

The Bad Cholesterol - LDL

Low-density lipoproteins are considered to be the bad cholesterol. The LDL cholesterol directly contributes to the buildup of fat in the arteries which is known as atherosclerosis. Having this condition causes the arteries to be narrowed. There is a direct connection between the narrowing of your arteries and the increased risk of strokes, heart attacks, heart disease, and peripheral artery disease, also known as PAD.

Having too much of this cholesterol in our bodies can be extremely harmful. Our best way to control how much of the bad cholesterol we have in our bodies is by controlling how much of the good cholesterol we have.

The Good Cholesterol – HDL

High-density lipoproteins can be considered the good cholesterol. Where with LDL we should have less of it in our bodies, with HDL we can argue that it's better that we have more of it.

Higher levels of HDL could help our bodies lower the levels of LDL. Experts in the subject have found evidence that HDL carries the LDL cholesterol from the arteries and back to the liver. Once it is there, the liver breaks down the LDL until it is passed from the body. However, HDL does not rid the body of all of the LDL cholesterol. HDL only carries about one-third to one-fourth of the LDL cholesterol in our blood to the liver. It cannot carry the remainder. There is evidence to suggest that having a higher HDL level can help protect us against things like heart attacks and strokes. Studies have also been done that show people with low levels of HDL are at a greater risk of heart disease.

Triglycerides

Having high levels of LDL or low levels of HDL cannot contribute to heart disease all by itself. Another thing that plays an important role are triglycerides. This is the most common type of fat we have in our body. What this fat does is it stores excess energy it gets from your diet. This fat is also linked to the risk of heart disease.

When you have a high level of triglycerides in your body combined with either a high level of LDL or a low level of HDL, you are at more risk of having a fatty buildup in your arteries. This is a direct link between this and heart attacks or strokes.

What You Need to Know About Cholesterol

Cholesterol is a waxy substance in your body that we all get from two sources. We get it from our liver, and from the food we eat. Cholesterol travels through our bodies in the bloodstream. It usually travels in fatty bundles known as lipoproteins.

We have low-density lipoproteins or LDL, which is the bad cholesterol. This kind of cholesterol can slow your blood flow, clog your arteries, and create blood clots. When your LDL levels are high, you are at a greater risk of heart attacks, strokes, and heart disease.

We also have high-density lipoproteins or HDL in our bodies, which is the good cholesterol. This type of cholesterol removes the bad cholesterol from your blood and takes it to your liver where it can be broken down and removed from the body. When your HDL levels are high you are at a lower risk of heart attacks, strokes, and heart disease.

That is the basic information that you need to know about cholesterol. Cholesterol is solely tied to the cause of heart disease, so it is targeted by doctors and medical professions. Although having the wrong levels of cholesterol in your body can raise your risk of heart disease, it isn't the only thing that can cause it. There are many other things that can increase the risk of heart disease in anyone. People tend to single out cholesterol as the main cause because it can be treated with drugs, diet, and exercise. However, most of the other things that can cause heart disease can also be easily controlled and countered.

Other Causes of Heart Disease

1: Smoking

This one is a no brainer, really. Smoke from cigarettes can give the body a lot of problems. One of those problems is raising the cholesterol. Not only does smoking raise your cholesterol levels, it also forces your heart to work harder. All of this puts you at risk of heart disease.

2: Obesity

It's not just obesity in general that can raise your risk of heart disease. To be more specific, it is the size of your waist that can raise your risk of heart disease. This is true even for people who have no previous risk of it.

3: Blood Pressure

It shouldn't come as a surprise that the higher your blood pressure is, the higher your risk of heart disease. When you have high blood pressure it can make your heart muscles stiff. There are a lot of things in life that can raise your blood pressure, but all of them can be controlled and eliminated as needed.

4: Diabetes

Diabetes is a problem all by itself and even if you're controlling your blood sugar levels, just the fact that you have diabetes raises your risk of heart disease.

5: Being Inactive

We need to be physically active in order to lower the risk of heart disease. Whether it's because of your job or your lifestyle, not everyone can be as physically active as they should be. When we exercise, we lower our blood pressure and help strengthen our hearts. So if we aren't getting enough exercise, then we weaken our hearts and raise our blood pressure which in turn raises our risk of heart disease.

6: Triglycerides

We've already discussed how this type of fat in our bodies is directly connected to heart disease. It's linked with cholesterol and this type of fat in your blood comes from the food you eat. Too much of it can cause a buildup in your arteries. We can control this by controlling how much of it we eat. Lowering the levels of this fat in our bodies will lower the risk of heart disease.

As you can see, there are far more causes of heart disease than just the cholesterol in our bodies. However, the big cholesterol myth will have you believe that the main and only cause of things like heart attacks and strokes is the level of cholesterol in your body. Nobody wants to tell you about the different types of cholesterol and why you need one type of it rather than just getting rid of all of it. It's easier for people to tell you to just cut down on the fat and lower your cholesterol levels, but it's far more complicated than that.

While all of the main causes of heart disease are somewhat controllable, there are some other causes that simply can't be controlled.

1: Age

There's no denying that the older you get, the more at risk you are of heart disease. Yes, there are things you can do to lower the risk as you get older. A good diet and active lifestyle lowers the risk at any age. However, as you get older, the risk will get higher and there's not much control over that.

2: Family History

We can't escape or control our history. Unfortunately, if your parents or grandparents had heart disease, then the chances that you'll have it as well are much higher. That's something that can't be controlled.

3: Gender

Yes, gender plays an uncontrollable factor in the risk of heart disease. If you're male you have a higher chance of having a heart attack at a young age. However, if you're female your risk of heart disease rises after menopause. Both men and women are at risk of heart disease, however men are at a greater risk at a young age than women are.

Controlling Your Cholesterol Levels

Here's what we know so far: among other things, having a high level of LDL cholesterol in your body or a low level of HDL cholesterol can put you at risk of heart disease. What we also know is that the levels of good and bad cholesterol in your body are directly connected to your diet. What we eat determines how high or low our cholesterol levels go. It's safe to assume that by controlling what we eat, we can lower our LDL levels and raise our HDL levels as we see fit.

You don't need your doctor to prescribe you any kind of drug. You don't need help from any of those money grabbing health and weight loss companies. All you need is to know what you're putting in your body and learn how to control your cholesterol levels.

Foods that Lower LDL Levels and Raise HDL Levels

One of the best ways to lower your LDL levels is to eliminate foods in your diet that have it. However, you can also add foods that counter the cholesterol and carry it out of the body in different ways. Some foods you can eat contain polyunsaturated fats; these are responsible for directly lowering LDL levels. Other foods combat it in a different way. Some have soluble fiber, which binds the LDL cholesterol in your digestive system so it is passed from the body before it even has the chance to enter the bloodstream. There are these and other ways that the food in your diet can help lower the LDL in your body.

1: Vegetable Oil

You can use oils like sunflower, canola, and other forms in place of things like lard or butter. These vegetables oils directly lower your LDL levels.

2: Oats

Oats or oat based foods contain a valuable ingredient, soluble fiber. Probably one of the easiest ways to lower your LDL levels is to have a bowl of oats or oat based cereal in the morning. It will give you 1 to 2 grams of soluble fiber a day.

3: Nuts

There are a lot of studies that show the benefits of nuts when it comes to your heart's health. All of these studies say that nuts are good for your heart, specifically peanuts, almonds, walnuts, and some others. If you eat at least 2 ounces of nuts a day, it can slightly lower your LDL levels.

4: Eggplants and Okras

These vegetables are a must have in any diet. They are low in calories and they contain soluble fiber which helps to directly lower LDL levels.

5: Strawberries, Citrus Fruits, Grapes, and Apples

These particular fruits are rich in pectin. Pectin is a type of soluble fiber which directly lowers your LDL levels. For your five fruits a day, make sure they're these fruits.

6: Whole Grains

Whole grains, like barley, are similar to oats. They can lower LDL levels in your body because they contain soluble fiber.

7: Fish

Adding fish to your diet, especially fatty fish, can help lower your LDL levels in multiple ways. One way is by replacing other meats with fish. Meat has saturated fats which boost LDL levels. If you eat fish a few times a week, you'd be replacing the LDL boosting meat and it will be giving you omega-3 which lowers LDL. Omega-3 does this by lowering the levels of triglycerides in your bloodstream.

8: Beans

Beans are useful for lowering LDL levels and for people who are trying to lose weight. Beans are rich in soluble fiber so they directly lower LDL. Beans also make you feel full faster so they are a must have in any weight loss diet.

9: High-fiber Fruits

Fruits that are high in fiber not only lower your LDL levels but they can also raise your HDL levels. Add fruits like pears and prunes to your diet in any way you want.

10: Avocados

This fruit isn't new on the scene of food, but it has gained recent popularity. It's high in fiber which naturally helps keep cholesterol levels in check and it contains a certain type of fat known as monounsaturated fat. This is a healthy fat and it can directly lower your LDL levels.

11: Red Wine

Yes you read that correctly. Red wine, when drunk in moderate amounts, can slightly raise your HDL levels. One glass of red wine a day for women and two glasses a day for men have been shown to lower the risk of heart disease among other benefits. This is a tricky one, though. You shouldn't just start drinking a glass a day straight away. The effectiveness of red wine is dependent on the other factors of your lifestyle. If you have high levels of triglycerides, then drinking red wine could actually do more harm than good. If this is the case, other drinks such as grape juice or just grapes can contain the same effects as red wine.

12: Soy Products

Soy products are mostly on the market for vegetarians but that doesn't mean that others can't eat them, too. If you add soy products to your diet, you can reduce the amount of meat you consume. We already know that meat can raise our cholesterol levels, so this is a good step to counter that. Although the fact that your HDL levels rise and your LDL levels lower is probably not directly connected to soy products, but rather as a result of eating soy instead of meat.

13: Chia and Flax Seeds

Flax seeds contain omega-3 and fatty acids. It's a favorite for vegetarians and helps to lower LDL levels in the body. Chia seeds are also a good source of omega-3 and are great for fiber. It directly lowers LDL levels and your blood pressure.

It's better to consume flax seeds once they are ground. If you eat them when they are whole, they won't be digested properly and your body won't absorb any of their nutrients. Chia seeds tend to gain a slimy texture once they are wet. If you don't want this, then rather consume them directly or add them to your baking.

Chapter 7:
Stop Counting Calories

Life is all about balance. Having a good and healthy lifestyle requires the perfect balance. For perfect balance we must understand what our bodies need and what we don't need. We must also understand that there is no good in eliminated something from our lives but we should rather try and see the good and bad of everything. There's no need to eliminate something completely when there is an option to only keep the good while removing the bad.

We've discussed the good and the bad in almost everything. Just like there are good and bad cholesterol, there are also good and bad calories. This, however, is not a widely known fact and that has harmed many people in many different ways.

The Calorie Myth

The current wide-spread method of weight loss is simple and easy to follow. All you have to do to burn fat and reach your goal weight is to eat less and exercise more. It sounds so easy that it's almost unbelievable. Well, that's because it doesn't work. This is an outdated and under studied method that has managed to squirm its way into society and for some reason hasn't been kicked out yet.

One of the most common low calorie diets is the 1200 calories a day diet. A lot of people are on this. They count calories religiously and exercise until they're sore every day. They do all this and yet for some people they don't see any results. In fact, many people work themselves to death eating less and exercising more just to lose weight but instead find themselves somehow gaining weight. This is because it isn't as simple as eating fewer calories, because not every calorie is the same. Most people dedicate their lives to managing their weight but if you don't actually know what the right thing to do is, then at the end of the day nothing you do will matter and that's the cold, hard truth.

The calorie myth states that all calories are equal and simply reducing your consumption of all of them will help you lose weight. By this logic, that means that if a glass of soda and a glass of freshly squeezed orange juice had the same amount of calories then it won't matter which glass you drink. Both glasses will have the same effect on you because they have the same amount of calories. This logic doesn't just sound ridiculous, it is ridiculous. It doesn't take an expert to realize that a glass of orange juice is far healthier than a glass of soda even if they contain the same amount of calories. This is the simple difference between good and bad calories.

The problem we find in diets, such as the 1200 calories a day diet, is that people on the diet are allowed to eat whatever they want as long as they stay in the allowed number of calories. Basically, someone could drink a glass of soda instead of orange juice because they'll still stay within their calorie limit. A person could stay under 1200 calories a day but it doesn't matter if all of the calories they're consuming are bad calories. The counting calories method is one bound for failure and there's no denying that.

There are of course other factors besides the fact that calories can be both good and bad. As mentioned before, the body needs to be perfectly balanced. It needs certain nutrients in order to function properly.

One of the main things in our bodies that assists us with weight loss is our metabolism. With a slow metabolism we're more likely to gain weight, and with a fast metabolism we're more likely to lose weight. In order to have a fast metabolism we need energy and we get that from food. If we starve ourselves of this food then we slow down our metabolism and ultimately gain more weight because of it. This is still connected to the difference between good and bad calories, of course. Certain foods can cause our metabolism to slow while other foods can speed it up.

In short, it doesn't matter that much how many calories we eat. What matters most is the type of calories we eat. We need to focus more on what we eat rather than on how much we eat. This is how your body works: when you eat more calories your body will automatically burn more calories, and when you eat fewer calories your body will automatically burn fewer calories. That's the simple science of it. It happens that way to everyone every time they go on a low calorie diet.

The 'calories in and calories out' system does still work to some extent. You can still end up overeating the good calories. Setting for yourself a calorie limit isn't exactly necessary, especially one so constrained as 1200 calories a day. However, you do need to set yourself some limits so you don't end up overeating.

The Importance of Quality over Quantity

Your body is like a system. It's like a machine and it has certain needs if you want it to keep running at an optimal rate. It's like a machine that runs on oil. The machine needs a certain amount of oil to run, and if it gets less oil than it needs it won't run properly. Your body needs a certain amount of calories in order to run properly. If it doesn't receive the correct amount, then it will slow down and eventually break down.

The problem with the modern world is that people don't change what they eat when they go on a low calorie diet. They simply eat less of it. They're still eating the same bad food but they make themselves feel better about it because they aren't eating a lot of it. That's what most people do and it is the first step on the path to disaster.

By eating less food we eventually end up starving our body of the food it needs to run properly. Once we do that we become hungry, tired to the point of lethargy, and we can even become depressed. This is a downward spiral. We can't keep this up forever. No one can essentially starve themselves forever. When we eventually crash we will not only stop eating less, we might even end up eating more than we were before we even started the diet. When this happens, and it will happen, you will end up not only gaining weight but you will gain more weight than you had before. This is the quantity over quality diet.

If your body requires a certain amount of calories to run properly, then it only makes sense that we feed our body that exact amount of calories. No more and no less. This way our bodies can run the way they're supposed to and give us the energy we need. It's not just about giving our bodies the correct amount of calories it needs. It's mostly about the kind of calories we give it.

There is evidence that by feeding our bodies the good calories, we help it heal itself. When we feed our body the correct calories it heals our brain, starts creating the correct hormones, and sets our gut back on the right track. When we heal our system we will start consuming and absorbing the right amount of calories and we will also start burning more of those calories. This all relies heavily on the type of food you give your body rather than the amount.

Protein is one of the best calories you can give your body for two beneficial reasons. The first reason is that protein fills you up better than other food groups. You'll end up eating about 100 calories of protein and you'll already feel full but if you eat

100 calories of carbohydrates, you'll still be hungry. The second and most beneficial reason you should eat protein is that it stops your body from burning muscle tissue instead of stored fat. When we reach the right amount of calories for our body to consume, our bodies will end up burning all of it. A big portion of the calories that our bodies burn comes from stored fat. If there isn't any stored fat for your body to burn it will start burning muscle tissue. This is very bad and you don't want this to happen. Adding protein to your diet can stop this from happening.

Protein is just one form of the good calories you can feed your body. You need to focus on the good food and how you can feed your body more of it. This is the quality over quantity diet.

Overall, it does matter how many calories you put into your body. However, the amount of calories doesn't matter nearly as much as the type of calories does. We can't starve our bodies of what they need. We need to at least give our bodies the exact number of calories it requires to run properly, no more and no less. Once we are only giving our body the calories it needs, it will end up burning up all of them and then some. This is why it is required that we are giving our body the good calories and not the bad. Then we can use smart exercise to fill in the rest of the gaps and speed up weight loss. The most important thing to remember out of all of this is if you want to lose weight, starving your body isn't the answer. Giving your body exactly what it needs is the right way to go about it.

Exercise Smart

Along with the calorie counting myth, we get the exercising more myth. People often say that you should eat less and workout more. They encourage you to work out every day and push yourself beyond your limits. While there is some truth in this, there is also a potential to hurt your body badly.

The main exercise options are aerobic exercises that are suitable for burning calories. These exercises include things like jogging daily. This is a good way to go about things, but there are better ways. Exercising smart involves low-impact but high-intensity exercises for about 20 minutes, up to once or twice a week. You can do more by exercising harder.

Most of the exercise advice that people have these days focuses primarily on burning calories. Burning calories isn't enough, though. Your body is already burning calories itself. The best exercises we can do involve trying to improve upon the calorie burning system we already have. The best and easiest way to do this is by building up our metabolism and adjusting our hormonal balance. We can do this through exercise as well as food.

We can achieve this by engaging all four of our muscle fibers during exercise. We have four types of muscle fibers. During an exercise such as jogging, we are only engaging one type of muscle fiber. In order to engage all four types of muscle fiber, we must produce more force for our bodies. This means that we need to exercise harder, move faster, and just have more intensity in our exercise routines. When we do this we won't have a need to exercise every day because you'll get quite a few days worth of exercise in just one day.

The reason we want to engage all four muscle fibers is because it will force our body to produce certain hormones. Our bodies will be forced to produce adrenaline, growth hormone, epinephrine, and noradrenaline. All of these hormones are clog-clearing hormones and they work to free up the energy that is being stored as body fat.

Your body naturally tries to use as little energy as possible when performing any given task. The muscle fiber's job is to conserve energy at all costs. If you lift something heavy, your body will use as little muscle fibers as possible to do so but if it sees that you require more muscle fibers, then it will give you more. It does this until eventually you end up using all four of your muscle fibers. You have to push your body past its comfort zone if you hope to use all of your muscle fibers. However, you don't want to do this the wrong way or you'll end up using too much energy which means you won't be able to exercise as much. That's where knowing how to exercise the smart way comes in handy.

Things like taking the stairs, going for a daily walk, or even a bike ride are all fine for general health and keeping active. These types of exercises generally work on your duration and frequency but they don't work on your resistance. The best chance you have of losing weight is to build up your resistance. You can accomplish this with targeted resistance training.

What you want to do is some high-intensity interval training for about 10 minutes, two times a week. That's all you need to do. Eccentric muscle workouts are the best because they leave your muscles feeling sore for a few days. You take those few days to rest, then once the sore feeling is gone you can exercise again. This will leave you about two days a week to exercise and if you're doing it right, that should be enough.

An eccentric workout is when your muscle is worked while it is lengthened. It's basically the opposite of lifting weights because all of eccentric workouts involve lowering weights. An eccentric movement is like when you're lowering your body into a squat or if you're lowering a dumbbell after you've lifted it. Studies show that during eccentric movement every muscle fiber in your body is at its strongest.

When you're exercising, make sure to do a full body workout. Get every single part of your body involved. People usually have leg days, arm days, and chest days. That works for some people, but to get the best results you have to get your whole body into it in one day. So work out your chest, legs, arms, back, shoulders, and abdominals all in one for the best possible workout.

Eating Smart

We've abolished the calorie myth. We've shown you that calories are not the same and that what you eat matters far more than how much you eat. Now we can talk about what you should be eating. It's all very well me telling you that you shouldn't eat bad calories, but how are you supposed to know what the good calories are? I won't leave you to guess. I can tell you what qualities a food must have if it falls into the category of good calories.

1: Nutrition

This is a given ingredient in any healthy food, or good calories. If a food can provide you with the nutrients you need, then it should be added to your diet. You want nutrients such as vitamins, essential amino acids, minerals, phytonutrients, and essential fatty acids. The more nutrients there are per calorie, the better.

Sweets, starchy foods, and sugary drinks usually have few nutrients if any and carry a lot of calories. Low-sugar fruits, nuts, protein, non-starchy vegetables, and seeds usually contain a lot of nutrients and fewer calories.

2: Satiety

If a food is able to make you feel fuller faster, then that is good for any diet. A food that makes us feel full has satisfied our appetite. There are many foods out there that don't satisfy our appetites and keep us eating more. Things like pizza do this. We will end up consuming a lot of calories without feeling full and this is a bad thing for anyone trying to lose weight.

Foods like broccoli, protein-rich meat, and tuna can make us feel full while not eating too many calories.

3: Non-aggressive

There are calories out there that trigger the production of glucose in our bodies. With the increased production of glucose, our body is more likely to store anything we're eating as body-fat. We call these aggressive foods. It's best to avoid the foods that do this and stick to the non-aggressive foods.

4: Digestibility

The harder it is for your body to digest a food, the better. If the body cannot efficiently digest a certain food, then it's less likely that food will be converted into stored body-fat. Our bodies can't digest fiber so it can't be stored as body-fat. Protein is also difficult for the body to digest; therefore it is passed through the body instead of being stored as body-fat. The body does try to digest these foods but after spending calories, so with little luck it eventually gives up on the food and it is passed. These foods are better to eat because they will cut down on the amount of body fat that is stored inside you.

Starches and sugars are usually easy to digest, so they are always stored as body fat. Fats are easily converted but they also have other desirable factors that make them a good addition to any diet, in moderation of course.

Chapter 8:
Eating to Prevent Cancer

When it comes to the risk of cancer, there are very few causing factors that we can control. Things like genetics are completely uncontrollable. If there is a history of cancer in your family, then you are at a greater risk of getting cancer yourself and there isn't much you can do about it unfortunately. However, some studies suggest that up to 70 percent of your risk of cancer throughout your life is within your control.

Avoiding known cancer causing products is fully within our control. Things like smoking cigarettes, drinking alcohol, exercising regularly, and keeping your body at a healthy weight are all under your control and making the right choices can lower your risk of cancer. Having the right diet can also lower your risk of cancer. We all know that there are foods out there that are known as cancer causing foods. There are also foods you can eat that can help you lower your risk of cancer.

What you eat or don't eat is a big part of your health, even to the point where it could lower your risk of cancer. Even if you have a history of cancer in your family, making small changes to your lifestyle can still lower your risk.

Red Meat and Processed Meat

For a few generations now red meat, such as pork, beef, and processed meats such as bacon and ham, have been labeled as cancer causing foods. This information has shaped the dietary guidelines and the pyramid of food since the beginning. The World Health Organization has classified red meat and processed meat as a Group 1 carcinogen. This basically means that it is known to cause cancer in people who consume certain amounts of it each day. Of course, this has not stopped the public from consuming these products. According to research, the average American diet consists of 4 and a half servings of red meat a week. Even more, about 10 percent of the population consumes two servings of red meat a day.

The science behind this information used to seem pretty solid. We were told that research showed that there were certain chemicals in processed and red meat that made the food carcinogenic. These chemicals were both natural and added during processing. According to this research, a chemical in red meat and processed meat known as haem is broken down in the gut once the food is consumed. When we break down this chemical, it forms other chemicals known as N-nitroso. The research showed that the N-nitroso chemical damages cells that line the bowel. This ultimately leads to bowel cancer. This research also suggested that the chemical was more present in processed meat than red meat and so processed meat should be avoided at all times. However, recent information has put doubt into this research. Recently, an international collaboration of researchers, through various trials and studies, found that this information which has shaped the American Dietary Guidelines for generations stands on shaky evidence.

The research involved looking through trials that linked red meat to cancer. The researchers also looked at articles that examined the links between red meat and incidence of cancer and mortality. Every study found that there were little to no links between red meat and disease or death. The quality of evidence that has been used to form the Dietary Guidelines was very low.

I should say that even though the links between red meat, processed meat, and cancer are low, they do still exist.

However, most of the research that has been done proving that red meat and processed meat cause cancer was done on large groups. In the region of science, evidence gained from large group studies is weak evidence. If a link was found in a few people amongst a large group, then how can they suggest that a single person will benefit from cutting out these products?

The evidence on both sides of this argument can be considered weak. However, even with knowing the risk of cancer that comes with eating these products, it hasn't stopped anyone. Red and processed meats are still a large part of the average American diet. Even if these products aren't the big cancer causers as we've been told all this time, it still wouldn't hurt to cut down on them.

Cancer Causing Foods

Red and processed meats have 'clogged up' the pool of cancer causing foods. Most of the talk about cancer causing foods has basically surrounded these two products, but there are several more that can share the same blame. Avoiding these foods and drinks altogether or limiting your consumption of them will reduce your risk of cancer.

There are so many articles and research papers out there telling you that they know what foods cause cancer. Everyone seems to have the facts. With there being so many facts out there, how are we supposed to determine which facts are true and which ones are false? We do it by looking at what we know. For a food to be labeled under cancer causing, it needs to be carcinogenic and for that to happen there has to be strong evidence that consumption of a food or drink can lead to an increased risk of cancer.

1: Alcohol

This is a given choice. There has been plenty of research and a lot of evidence to prove that alcohol causes cancer. To be specific, the more alcohol you drink, the greater your risk is of contracting head, liver, breast, neck, colorectal, and esophageal cancer.

When we drink alcohol it produces a chemical compound known as acetaldehyde. This chemical compound may cause damage to your DNA and this is what leads to the risk of cancer.

Although it's better to avoid alcohol altogether, experts have come up with an allowable daily limit. That is one serving of alcohol a day for women and two for men. Serving sizes vary depending on the type of alcohol. A serving of wine would be 5 oz., beer is 12 oz., and liquor is 1.5 oz.

2: Diet food and drinks

Diet foods and drinks have gained popularity at an alarming rate. They're supposed to be a better and healthier way for us to enjoy some of our favorite guilty pleasures. Recent studies have shown that certain diet foods and drinks may not be as healthy we are lead to believe.

Diet foods and drinks are made with the use of artificial sweeteners. This eliminates the use of the harmful refined sugar but adds something even more harmful. The European Food Safety Authority has done up to 20 separate studies that found one of the most commonly used artificial sweeteners, aspartame, as the cause of a range of illnesses including cancer. There are various other sweeteners that have been linked to the cause of cancer, such as saccharin and sucralose.

Diet foods and drinks are dangerous and they don't really do that much for our health. It's best to avoid them completely.

3: Refined Sugars

While you're avoiding diet foods and drinks, it's also best to avoid refined sugar products as well. There are multiple reasons to avoid refined sugar. One of the main reasons is that it tends to spike your insulin levels, which in turn feeds cancer cells. Fructose-rich products such as high fructose corn syrup or HFCS is probably the most harmful. Studies have shown that cancer cells can easily and quickly metabolize HFCS in order to spread. Sodas, cereals, cookies, pies, cakes, juices, sauces, and other processed products have a lot of HFCS in them along with other forms of refined sugar. These are popular products that are filled with cancer causing ingredients.

4: GMOs

GMOs or genetically-modified organisms and the chemicals that are used to grow them have been proven to contribute to the rapid growth of tumors. GMOs are in basically everything. The only way to properly avoid them is to stick with certified organic, locally grown food, and non-GMO verified foods. Try to buy foods that are produced naturally.

5: Microwave Popcorn

Placing a bag in the microwave for a few minutes for a nice snack may seem convenient, but it is also more harmful than you would think. The bags of microwave popcorn are lined with chemicals such as perfluorooctanoic or PFOA. This chemical has been linked to the cause of testicular, liver, and pancreatic cancer. There are several independent studies proving the chemical causes tumors. There is another chemical in popcorn known as diacetyl that is linked to lung damage and eventually lung cancer.

6: 'Dirty' Fruit

Dirty fruit is basically any food that is verified and certified organic and pesticide-free. You may think that you're being healthy by buying that bag of apples or grapes, but for all you know they are covered in pesticides which are cancer causing chemicals. Conventional produce is a no go. Studies have found that up to 98 percent of conventional produce are covered with these cancer causing pesticides. It's best to make sure your fruits are organic and verified pesticide-free.

7: Refined White Flour

Refined flour is commonly used in a lot of processed foods. The worrying thing about this ingredient is the excess amount of refined carbohydrates in it. A recent study that was published in the Cancer Epidemiology journal showed that refined carbohydrates, like those found in refined flour, are linked to an increase in the risk of breast cancer. This was a significant increase of 220 percent. Foods that are high-glycemic have been proven to raise blood sugar levels. Something like this directly feeds cancer cells and helps them grow and spread.

8: Soda Pops

Soda pops are generally unhealthy, as they are loaded with many forms of refined sugar. They're also filled with food chemicals and colorings. Soda pops directly feed cancer cells and they acidify the body. The most common chemicals used in soda pops such as caramel color and 4-methylimidazole are also directly linked to causing cancer.

9: Hydrogenated Oil

Hydrogenated oil is mostly used in processed foods as a preservative. The use of hydrogenated oil allows companies to extend the shelf life of their processed products. However, this ingredient has been linked to altering the structure and flexibility of cell membranes. This can raise the risk of many diseases including cancer.

Recently, a few companies have made steps to fade out the use of hydrogenated oil, but trans fats are still used in processed food and it isn't that much better.

10: Farmed Salmon

Farmed salmon is a high risk cancer food as it is loaded with chemicals in order to lengthen its shelf life. It lacks vitamin D which is something you should get from fish such as salmon. It's also often contaminated with pesticides, flame retardants, antibiotics, and polychlorinated biphenyls or PCB. All of these chemicals are carcinogenic. Avoid farmed fish at all cost and buy fresh, because fish is a really good addition to any diet as long as it isn't contaminated with chemicals.

11: Sugar

Sugar is loosely implicated as a cause of certain kinds of cancers. Otto Warburg, a German biochemist, found that cancer cells often used sugar to fuel their growth. This study was done in the early 20th century. The Warburg effect, which was established after his discovery, suggests that if you starve the body of sugar and things that can be converted into sugar like carbohydrates, then you could in turn starve the cancer cells. This is how the ketogenic diet was created. This diet reduces the amount of carbohydrates you consume to about 10 percent. It also increases your fat consumption by 70 percent. This supposedly works to slow down and starve the cancer cells. However, the effectiveness of this diet has not been scientifically proven to help slow down cancer cells and it comes with a lot of other health problems if not done properly.

The association between the increased risk of cancer and sugar is still there. It could help to cut down your consumption of sugar. When most people do this they tend to replace sugar with artificial sweeteners which have the same effect as sugar. Both of them should be avoided or taken in moderation if at all possible.

12: Very Hot Drinks

It sounds strange, but it's true. The evidence for it is sparse but it is there. Studies have been done that show drinking hot beverages, such as tea and coffee, can raise your risk of esophageal cancer. However, you don't have to cut these beverages out of your diet. You just need to wait for them to cool down first. If your beverage is hotter than 140 degrees Fahrenheit, or 60 degrees Celsius, then it is putting you at risk of cancer. Any temperature lower than that should be perfectly fine.

The reasons for a hot beverage to increase our chances of getting cancer are unclear. The evidence is there, but the exact cause is still unknown. It's believed that the raised risk in cancer may be linked to the damaged caused by the heat blanching our throat's cells.

Don't let this information put you off drinking any hot beverages. In fact, certain types of tea are good for your health and can even help you lower your risk of cancer. All you have to do to safely enjoy these beverages is wait for them to cool down before drinking them.

13: Burnt or Charred Food

Meat or food that is cooked at too high a temperature, burnt, or charred can raise your risk of cancer. If you burn your toast, you could be raising your risk of contracting cancer. If you like your meat well-done or barbecued, then you could also be increasing your risk. When meats are cooked at high temperatures or cooked to the point where they are burnt or charred, they start to form chemicals that may change your DNA when you eat it. This can lead to a higher chance of getting cancer.

If you are used to eating a large amount of meat that is fried, well-done, barbequed, or even slightly charred, then you are raising your risk of pancreatic, prostate, and colorectal cancer.

You can avoid this by slow cooking your meat at a low temperature. You could also bake, boil, or braise your meat instead. Some evidence has shown that marinating your meat before you cook it could help lower your risks.

Making these small changes to your diet can lower your chances of contracting any kind of cancer significantly. Some foods should be removed from your diet altogether, while other foods should be eaten in moderation. The key to any well balanced diet is moderation.

Cancer Preventing Foods

Just like there are foods that can increase your risk of cancer, there are also foods that could lower your risk. You can eat your way to health and to a low risk of a variety of cancers. For example, a traditional Mediterranean diet could help lower your risk for many different kinds of cancer. This diet is rich in vegetables, fruits, olive oil, and healthy fats. These foods are on the list of foods that lower your risk. Even if you have a history of cancer in your family, you can still lower your risk by changing your lifestyle for the better.

Of course, there are other factors involved in the prevention of cancer, such as lifestyle, body weight, and how active you are. However, you can change your risk by a small amount just by changing your diet. You should still try to change your whole lifestyle for the better, as it will increase your chances of cancer prevention by a much more significant amount.

1: Fruits and Vegetables

It's recommended that we all eat at least five different fruits and vegetables a day. I think I speak for everyone when I say that not all of us manage to reach this limit. However, adding a variety of farm fresh, natural fruits and vegetables to our diet can help better our health in many different ways, including lowering the risk of cancer. I am, of course, talking about what we call whole foods. For example, a whole, unpeeled apple is far healthier than apple juice.

These are certified natural, fresh, and verified pesticide and preservative free. All of those chemicals are used to preserve the food's shelf life but, as we've already discussed, they also raise our chances of contracting cancer.

Once you've managed to find fruits and vegetables that fall under the whole food category, then you can add them to every aspect of your diet.

Add fresh cut fruit to your cereal in the morning. You can add cut fruit to your oatmeal, or Greek yogurt for a nice healthy start to the day. For lunch you can have fruit as a side or even some raw vegetables. A salad packed with vegetables with a side of fruit is extremely healthy. If you have snacks during the day, then make it a fruit or raw vegetables. And for dinner, you can fill your plate with fresh or frozen vegetables. Make sure at least half of your plate is made up of veggies.

2: Healthy Fats

It's been proven that having a diet high in fat can raise your risk of contracting cancer. However, just like almost everything else, there are good fats and bad fats. While the bad fats can raise your risk of cancer and leave you unhealthy in many other ways, the healthy fats can help to lower your risk of cancer.

Trans fat should be avoided at all costs and saturated fats should be limited as much as possible. Unsaturated fats should be added to your diet and used in moderation. Unsaturated fats are the healthy fats and you can find them in olive oil, avocados, nuts, and fish. Omega-3 is a fatty acid and it is one of the healthiest unsaturated fats you can add to your diet. You can find an abundance of it in tuna, salmon, and flaxseeds.

3: Antioxidants

A diet high in antioxidants can help lower your risk of various cancers. It's mostly plant based foods where you'll find an abundance of nutrients known as antioxidants. These help to boost your immune system which protects from many diseases, including cancer.

You'll mostly find antioxidants in fruits and non-starchy vegetables, but there are other foods that carry them too. Keep your eye out for foods with this nutrient and add them to your diet.

4: Fiber

Fiber is a key ingredient to keeping your digestive system properly clean and healthy. A diet that contains fiber can help keep cancer causing compounds from moving through your digestive tract and stop them from doing any harm. Fiber can be found in several food groups but it's mostly found in fruits, vegetables, and whole grain foods.

5: Green Tea

Green tea is a tasty beverage and it's good for many different health problems. Green tea is especially useful as part of an anti-cancer diet. The reason is because it's a powerful antioxidant. Research has found a chemical called epigallocatechin-3 gallate in green tea. This is a non-toxic chemical that acts directly against an enzyme called urokinase which is a crucial ingredient for cancer cells to grow.

Green tea is a known cancer fighting food and it can help you fight against breast, lung, liver, pancreatic, skin, and esophageal cancer. Add a cup of green tea to your daily routine because just one cup contains 100 to 200 milligrams of this cancer fighting chemical.

6: Garlic and Onions

Garlic and onions are not world-wide favorite foods. In fact, they're more of an acquired taste and if they are used, they're used sparingly. However, you should consider using them as abundantly as possible. Research has shown that onions and garlic are able to block the formation of nitrosamines. Nitrosamines are powerful carcinogens that are able to target multiple parts of the body.

The chemically active sulfur compounds in garlic and onions can help you fight against colon, breast, and liver cancer. So don't just add them to your diet, add as much of them as possible. The more you add, the stronger your defense against the cancer cells.

7: Tomatoes

Lycopene, a type of antioxidant, is a powerful cancer fighting food and tomatoes contain a lot of it. Research has shown that this type of antioxidant is even more powerful than vitamin E, beta-carotene, and alpha-carotene which are all cancer fighting foods. Eating tomatoes can help protect against certain cancers such as lung cancer and prostate cancer. Make sure to cook the tomatoes before you eat them, as this helps release the Lycopene and makes it easy for your body to access.

8: Olive Oil

Olive oil is a monounsaturated fat, which is a healthy fat, and it is widely used in Mediterranean countries for cooking and as a salad dressing. Recent research has shown that the risk for breast cancer in Mediterranean countries is 50 percent lower than in other countries where olive oil is not as widely used. The evidence that makes this a cancer fighting food isn't as strong as with other foods, but it's worth adding it to your diet anyway.

9: Cinnamon

Cinnamon is well known across the world for its many health benefits. One of those health benefits includes blocking the spread of cancer cells. There have been several tube-tests and animal studies that show how cinnamon and cinnamon essential oil helps to prevent the spread and growth of cancer cells as well as reduce the size of tumors. One animal study showed that cinnamon extract caused cell death in tumor cells. This is how it managed to decrease growth and spread rate of the tumors.

Most of these studies that show cinnamon as being a helpful cancer fighting food have been done on animals and in test-tubes. There haven't been any studies done on humans that can prove its effectiveness on cancer cells in humans. However, it wouldn't hurt to add a teaspoon or so to your daily diet. It may be beneficial in not only preventing cancer but also decreasing inflammation, and reducing blood sugar levels.

10: Nuts

There have been several studies done on groups of people that could prove a link between eating nuts regularly and having a lower risk of cancer. One study followed 30,708 people for about 30 years. Every one of them was eating nuts regularly and the study found that it led to a decreased chance of contracting pancreatic, colorectal, and endometrial cancer.

Out of all the studies that have been performed, many of them have shown a positive link between nuts and their ability to prevent cancer. Brazil nuts, for example, contain a high amount of selenium. This chemical could help prevent lung cancer in people who have a low amount of selenium.

Although more studies need to be done on humans to solidify the evidence, it wouldn't hurt to add at least one serving of nuts to your daily diet.

11: Red Grapes

Grapes are on the list of healthy fruits you should add to your diet. Red grapes in particular carry a chemical known as superantioxidant activin which can mostly be found in their seeds. This chemical is a known cancer fighting chemical that can also be found in red wine. You can eat red grapes as a snack or eat them as regularly as you want. They can help protect against certain types of cancer as well as heart disease.

12: Whole Grains

Whole grains contain both fiber and antioxidants which are both proven to be cancer fighting chemicals. It wouldn't hurt to add a few whole grain foods to your diet.

Tips for Further Cancer Prevention

- Wash all of your fruits and vegetables before you eat them. This will reduce the risk of eating any pesticides or other residue.

- Try eating some raw fruits and vegetables. Don't just cook everything. The raw food will have more vitamins and minerals available for your body.

- Don't cook oils or meats on high heat. Slow cooking and baking on low heat are far healthier and cancer preventing than cooking everything on a high heat. Avoid cooking anything, including meat and oil, on high heat.

- Instead of frying or sautéing your foods, try the healthier cooking options such as boiling, steaming, baking, or broiling.

- Store all of your oils in cool dark places and make sure they are in airtight containers.

- Be wary when using the microwave. Always use microwave safe containers or waxed paper when covering something in the microwave.

- Avoid anything that looks or smells like it might be moldy. It will mostly likely contain aflatoxin which is a carcinogen. It's mostly found on moldy peanuts.

- When you cook your vegetables, try only steaming them until they are tender. This will preserve as much of their vitamins and minerals as possible.

By following the correct diet and a healthy, active lifestyle, you can significantly lower your risk of contracting various types of cancer. Remember that everything is good in moderation. Even the good, healthy foods should be eaten in moderation. There is such a thing as too much of a good thing.

Chapter 9:
Carbs Don't Fuel Your Brain

There is a game that children like to play. I'm sure we've all played it at one point when we were younger. This game is called telephone. What this game proves is that if information is passed down through too many mouths and too many ears it gets twisted, mixed up, and changed until eventually the new information is nothing like the original information. This may be a fun and amusing game for children to play, but unfortunately it is also one of the main problems we get in the medical industry.

Information is passed from doctor to doctor, from nutritionist to nutritionist, and from patient to patient until eventually the information is turned into untrue rumors or myths that have become extremely dangerous to the public's general health. The brain fuel myth is one such instance of this happening. This myth has convinced people that the brain uses carbohydrates to fuel itself. It has encouraged people to eat a high carb diet in order to fuel their brains, but a high carb diet is unhealthy and harmful in many ways and it does not fuel our brains. This is a just another myth that has been used to line the pockets of the industry.

The brain is a very complicated thing. It's like the world's most complicated computer. It's so complicated that a human brain can't even understand a human brain. It's probably one of the most important and complicated organs in our bodies, and yet there are people out there who think they understand how it works. People like this are the reason we have such a myth as this one. Do carbohydrates fuel your brain, or are they actually bad for you? This probably looks like a simple question that should have a simple answer. However, with everyone out there fighting to be the one that knows the right answer, how can you trust any answer that is given to you?

People are now convinced that we need at least 130 grams of carbohydrates a day for our brains to function normally. This is for both adults and children. They say that if you restrict carb consumption you are effectively starving your brain. Even the largest diabetes charity organization in the world, the American Diabetes Association or ADA, says that, "The recommended dietary allowance (RDA) for digestible carbohydrates is 130 grams per day." However, none of these people actually state why we need so many carbs a day. Sure they say that the carbs fuel our brains, but where is the evidence? How do the carbs help our brains to function? No one seems to know the answer to that question. Or do they? The ADA also says, "Providing adequate glucose as the required fuel for the central nervous system." Now we have our answer! It's not 130 grams of carbs we need, its 130 grams of glucose per day that fuels our brains.

Carbs can be converted by the body into glucose, but so can fat and protein. Protein is slow and inefficient for the body to convert into glucose, so fat is probably the better choice.

How Does the Brain Work?

The brain is the hungriest organ in your body. It takes up about 2 percent of your body weight, but it ends up using 50 percent of your body's glucose and about 20 percent of your body's oxygen. It's considered to be one of the more greedy organs.

When it comes to feeding your brain, it likes to burn glucose for food. It very rarely looks to anything else for fuel. Your brain spends 99 percent of your waking life operating on glucose. It's designed that way. When the brain doesn't get the glucose it needs, the results can be disastrous. If you suffer from low blood sugar or diabetes, then you've probably experienced hypoglycemia. This is what happens when your brain is starved. It results in blurry vision, slurred speech, lightheadedness, and a loss of balance. It can lead to effects far more dangerous that these as well.

The brain is designed to use only glucose as fuel. When the glucose levels in our bloodstream drop for any reason, the brain is the first organ to notice. When your brain isn't getting the amount of glucose it needs, it is literally being starved. Along with the above symptoms of a starved brain, it can also eventually lead to fatality. This is why we need glucose in our bodies and this is also why the rumor that our brains need carbohydrates has spread so far.

The Source of Glucose

We know that our brains need glucose to function. What we don't know is how to efficiently get that glucose into our bodies. A study done on women in 2008 showed that women who were on a low-carbohydrate diet suffered several effects on their brains. These effects included impaired reaction time and reduced spatial memory. Women who were placed on a high-carbohydrate diet, however, did not suffer any of these effects. This research has led scientists and nutritionists to tell the public that they need to feed their bodies carbs in order to provide the right amount of glucose that their brains need.

What we aren't told is that there are other ways for your body to get what it needs. The body is like a well-oiled machine and the brain is the computer that runs it. If something is missing that is needed, the brain and body will work together to find a way to get what it needs. The same happens when the brain is in need of glucose.

There are groups of people, such as the Eskimos, who live solely on a meat-rich diet and eat little to no carbohydrates. Yet these people do not suffer any effects on their brain. The brain cannot survive without glucose. That means that the Eskimos must be getting the glucose they need from a source other than carbs.

When someone goes on a low-carb diet or one that has no carbs, their brain will quickly realize that there isn't enough glucose in the bloodstream. It doesn't take long for the situation to be solved. At this point the brain and liver will quickly work together to find another source of energy. The liver realizes it can convert other sources of food into the fuel that the brain needs. The liver can convert protein into glucose and then send it straight to the brain for immediate use. However, protein is slow and inefficient to convert, so the liver makes up for this by converting fat into something called ketone bodies and sends them up to the brain as an alternative source of energy. Your brain is able to quickly adapt to this new source of fuel and uses it as it is given.

Instead of blindly believing that our brains need carbohydrates to function, we can look at the facts and realize that what we actually need is glucose and there is more than one source for that.

Ketone Bodies

Ketone bodies are a secondary fuel source for our brains when there isn't enough glucose available. It's like having a backup battery for your phone. These are backup power sources for the brain. Ketone bodies are created easily when we are on a high protein and high fat diet. These are the building blocks for our brain's backup energy source.

The reason that people aren't aware of this is because the switch from glucose to ketone bodies is not immediate. The liver can react to the lack of glucose in the body quickly but it will take a while for the brain and the body to adapt. This is why the change is usually so painful and why most people who try to go low-carb usually give up. The transition from running on glucose to running on ketone bodies is approximately 2 weeks. It takes 2 weeks for your body to fully adapt to using this alternative fuel source rather than the one it is used to. After the transition period your body and brain will not only function properly but some research shows that the brain will actually be more efficient on ketone bodies than it is on glucose.

Another advantage of the use of ketone bodies is that they last longer. Once the brain has adapted to using ketone bodies for fuel it is able to function longer on them than it could on glucose only. A brain run completely on ketone bodies can function for weeks, months, or even years on a low amount of them.

Carbohydrates versus Fat and Protein

The Carbohydrate myth has led people to believe that they need 130 grams of carbs a day for their brains to function properly. The truth is that your body actually needs 130 grams of glucose a day. Carbohydrates are a source of glucose, but they aren't the only source. As we discussed, the body finds a way to make glucose out of protein and ketone bodies out of fat. Both of these can be used as a fuel source by our brains. We know all this, but still there is an argument as to whether we should fuel our brains with carbs or ketone bodies.

The Eskimos have proven that an all meat diet doesn't harm the brain and it actually provides them with excellent health. There is evidence to support that our brains function perfectly fine without carbs and some of our brains may even function better on a low-carb diet. There is also similar evidence that supports carbohydrates as fuel for our brains. With so much evidence supporting both low and high carbohydrate diets, it's hard to choose what is best for your own brain's functions.

When it comes to this, I guess all I can say is that the choice is up to you. The brain can function both with and without carbohydrates. All you have to decide is which diet you prefer. There are other advantages that come with a low-carb diet as well as some disadvantages. Being able to make the right choice for the health of both your body and your brain means knowing exactly what kind of life you want to live and what kind of life you can actually afford to live.

Chapter 10:
Viruses and Antibiotics

Recently there has been an epidemic of inappropriately prescribed antibiotics and an overuse of antibiotics as well. Most patients aren't even aware of what an antibiotic is used for or why they're being prescribed it. Along with the instances of inappropriately prescribed antibiotics, there are also instances where antibiotics aren't being used properly. All of this has led to what is called an antibiotic resistance.

What are Antibiotics?

An antibiotic is a powerful drug that is used to treat certain illnesses. It is a very powerful medicine and can be very dangerous if used inappropriately. Antibiotics, as powerful as they are, cannot be used to treat everything. They should only be prescribed to people who have certain infections.

There are only two types of infections a person can get. Here are some examples of the two:

Viral Infections:

1. Colds

2. Flus

3. Sore Throats

4. Coughs and Bronchitis

5. Runny noses

6. Some ear or eye infections

7. Acute sinusitis

8. Respiratory Syncytial Virus (RSV)

Bacterial Infections:

1. Urinary tract infections

2. Ear infections

3. Strep throat

4. Sinus infections

Antibiotics are prescribed to people with bacterial infections and they should be used for this only. Certain antibiotics are used for certain bacterial infections. An antibiotic cannot be used to cure a viral infection. Viral infections are usually left for your body to cure by itself and an antibiotic should never be used to cure a viral infection.

In some instances a doctor won't know whether they should prescribe their patient antibiotics or not. Some viruses can cause a patient to have the same symptoms that would resemble a bacterial infection. This is where the problem comes in. The doctor can tell the patient that they have a viral infection and not prescribe them any antibiotics. However, the patient may return later after their symptoms worsen and the doctor will realize that they had a bacterial infection and they need antibiotics. At this point it may be too late to prescribe simple antibiotics as the infection could be too bad. Likewise, a doctor can diagnose their patient with a bacterial infection and prescribe them antibiotics when really they only had a viral infection. Not only do the antibiotics do nothing for the viral infection, they also cause the patient to suffer bad side effects and grow an antibiotic resistance.

Why Can't Antibiotics Kill Viruses?

You can think of bacteria and viruses as types of machines. They work through all of the small, intricate parts of

95

machinery. Viruses have a different structure than bacteria. They are two completely different machines.

Antibiotics are designed to target the part of the machinery that helps the bacteria grow. It does this so it can kill or inhibit that particular type of bacteria. It can't do the same thing with viruses because viruses are built differently and use a different type of machine to grow and replicate.

The machinery that helps the bacteria to replicate and grow is completely different than the machinery that a virus uses to replicate and grow. Therefore, because the antibiotic is designed to target the bacteria's type of machinery, it wouldn't be able to do the same to a virus's machinery. With a virus, the antibiotic won't have a target to attack.

If you try to cure a virus with an antibiotic, here is what will happen:

1. You will not cure the virus and no relief from the symptoms will be provided.

2. You won't feel better and you may even feel worse.

3. You will probably end up with some bad side effects.

4. You'll build up a resistance to antibiotics.

5. You won't prevent other people from catching your virus.

6. You'll be wasting your money and your time.

Antibiotic Resistance and Resistant Bacteria

Antibiotic Resistance and Resistant Bacteria are very big issues that are beginning to arise of late. They are a big threat to global health. In fact, the US Centers for Disease Control and Prevention say that it is one of their top concerns at the moment.

Antibiotic resistance happens when a bacteria gains the ability to withstand the effects of a certain antibiotic. Basically, when once an antibiotic was used to cure a certain bacterial disease the next time it is used, it could be less effective or have no effect at all against the bacteria.

The main reason for the current rise in antibiotic resistance is the overuse of antibiotics. Antibiotics are being prescribed by doctors when they aren't needed and people aren't being properly instructed on how to use them. Another cause of antibiotic resistance comes from patients not finishing their trial of antibiotics. Patients are prescribed enough antibiotics for a certain amount of time. Sometimes they stop taking them early simply because they feel better. It doesn't matter if you feel better, your body still needs to finish the trial of antibiotics. If you don't finish all of them, then you could be adding to the bacteria's resistance to it.

There is a misconception that our bodies are becoming resistant to the antibiotics. This is just another one of those myths. Our bodies are not becoming resistant, the bacteria itself is becoming resistant.

Lately people are discussing the existence of superbugs. These are bacterial infections that have become completely resistant to any known antibiotic that we have available to us. Records state that every year at least 2 million people contract a bacterial infection that is antibiotic resistant and almost 23,000 of them die from this infection.

You're probably wondering how the bacteria are able to become resistant to our antibiotics. It does this by adapting its structure in a defensive way. It can adapt in several ways; the bacteria can learn to pump the antibiotic out of the cells. It can share its genetic material with other bacteria in order to make them resistant as well. It can neutralize the effects of the antibiotic before it is able to kill the bacteria. The resistant bacteria then survive the effects of the antibiotics and are able to spread and cause further infections. Once it spreads, the new infections are resistant to the antibiotic that was used on them or any other similar antibiotics. The only way to combat this infection is with a completely new and stronger antibiotic.

Don't Take Them if You Don't Need Them

Another factor to the rising bacteria resistance epidemic, as I've already mentioned before, is the use of antibiotics when they are not needed. Some people will take an antibiotic 'just in case' if they're feeling under the weather. This is dangerous and a waste of both time and money. Taking them without needing them can also put you at risk of side effects. Some of them won't be harmful, like a rash, but some can be very harmful.

Taking antibiotics when you don't need them can also speed up the resistance to that antibiotic. This means that by the time you actually need to use them, they won't work anymore. In any case, you shouldn't have leftover antibiotics that you can take whenever.

When you're prescribed a certain amount of antibiotics, you're supposed to take all of them. If you don't finish them, even if you feel better, you don't completely kill the bacteria. A part of it is allowed to survive inside of you and that helps it become resistant to the antibiotics. Then the bacteria will come back stronger, it will hit you harder, and it will be more difficult to kill.

The best way we ourselves can combat bacterial resistance is by finishing our trial of antibiotics and by only taking them when we are told by a doctor that we actually need them.

Curing Viral and Bacterial Infections Correctly

Using antibiotics shouldn't be that complicated, but you'd be surprised by how many people actually use them incorrectly. It's possible to forget to take them when you're supposed to. That's natural human error. However, there are plenty of other errors that people make when it comes to antibiotics when they really should know better.

Here are a few things to keep in mind when dealing with antibiotics and any kind of infection:

1. We've already discussed the fact that you have to finish your antibiotic trial. There are no if's or but's about this one. You have to finish them.

2. The antibiotics that are prescribed to you are for you only. Your doctor chose that specific antibiotic to combat your specific bacterial infection. You can't give them to someone else who has an infection. Yes, you may have the best intentions at heart but in the end you're doing more harm than good to both of you. You're given a specific amount of antibiotics for a reason. You need all of them. Even if you only give one away, that's still one that you need to take in order to fully kill the bacteria. Your bacterial infection could be completely different in structure than their bacterial infection. Even if you have the same symptoms, there is no guarantee that your antibiotics will be able to combat their specific bacterial infection. Not only will you be putting them at risk of some bad side effects, but you probably won't be helping them at all. So, whatever you do make sure you finish all of your antibiotics and never give them to someone else.

3. A cold or flu cannot be treated or cured by an antibiotic. These are viral infections and antibiotics are useless

against them. Keep in mind that a viral infection does have the ability to grow and mutate into a bacterial infection. Because of this, people often take antibiotics to try and stop the bacterial infection before it has a chance to form. This doesn't work, it will give you harmful side effects, and if your viral infection does eventually become a bacterial infection there is a high chance that bacteria will already be resistant to the antibiotic you've been taking. Don't use any antibiotics if you have a viral infection. Rather, wait until your doctor is sure it's grown into a bacterial infection and gives you the antibiotics you need.

4. A viral infection is usually left to the body to cure. You can take drugs to relieve some of the symptoms but usually all you need is rest, fluids, and some time to recover. This is the only way to cure a viral infection. Let your body do what it does best and don't mess up your health.

5. Normally, with a bacterial infection, you should just take your antibiotics as prescribed and wait. There are a few things you can do to help boost your immune system so it has a better chance at fighting the infection. Some research has shown that giving your body healthy fibers along with taking your antibiotics can help your body protect itself against the bacterial infection. The antibiotics usually attack the infection directly. The fiber can help make your body strong so it can protect itself while the antibiotics work to attack the infection.

Any other questions you have should be answered by your doctor, but it's up to you to ask the questions. Most people aren't given the information they need because they don't ask for it. If you are willing to ask the questions, your doctor will answer them.

Conclusion

To conclude this book, I will leave you with one final message. Don't be afraid to take action. The problem out there is real. We are being manipulated and controlled by these big industries. Our lives have been taken out of our hands and placed in the hands of greedy businessmen. That's what the medical industry has become, a world of business and profit.

We don't have to sit down and take it. We can stand up and grab our lives right out of those greedy hands. You'll see once you start asking your doctors those hard questions they'll cave in. They'll admit they have no idea what you're talking about or they'll avoid the subject altogether just to save face. It's not only our job to ask the questions, it's also our responsibility to seek out the right answers. After all, our lives are our own and we should take responsibility for them.

You may be sitting there, marveling over everything I've told you, and you may be wondering, "What can I take away from this book?" Well that's good, because I want you to ask questions. Here is the answer:

Don't trust anything anyone tells you. Whether they're a doctor, a pharmacist, part of a weight loss and diet program, or part of the food industry. You can never fully trust anything they tell you. If they try to tell you what is what, challenge them. Ask them for more information and then take all of that information and poke holes in it. Whatever is left can be taken as a half-truth or full truth as you wish.

As I mentioned all the way at the beginning of the book, please don't take this information and use it as an excuse to forsake your doctors. They do know what they're talking about when it comes to some things and we do need them. We just don't have to fully trust them with our lives. Listen to what he has to say, just don't put all of your hope and faith into every word he says.

Not everything they say is bad for you is just bad for you. There aren't just bad calories and bad cholesterol. There are both good and bad of everything. There are good and bad calories and there are good and bad carbohydrates. The current lies and myths in the world of health will lead you to believe that you need to cut out these things altogether, but you don't. You only need to cut out the bad things and keep the good things. Your body needs calories and cholesterol, but it only needs the good kind. Keep that in mind.

Our health is under our control. We don't always have to rely on medicine and prescription drugs to maintain our body's health. We can control it through our diet and lifestyle. The things we eat can help us to lose weight, feel better, and they can even help us put off illnesses and lower our risk of cancer. We must always remember that even though sometimes medicine is needed to cure us, we can still do our part to feel better through proper diet and lifestyle.

It's good to remember there are a lot of myths out there. There's the cholesterol myth, the myth that your brain needs carbs, and of course the calorie myth. It's not just enough to know that these are myths. We need to be able to see through any other myths that we might encounter. We should always be willing to seek the truth ourselves and never just settle for what we're told. There are a lot of myths out there, some that I've told you about and some that are slowly making their way to the surface. Being able to spot a myth is a very valuable skill.

Now, I am confident that you are ready to restart your life for the better. You should be too. You've taken the necessary steps towards a better diet, and a better lifestyle. You should be proud of yourself. I promised I would lead you down the right path and here we are, at the end of the road. All that you have learned will guide you from now on. You don't need me anymore. Don't hesitate. You've started the ball rolling and you need to keep it that way. If you let the ball stop it might be more difficult to get it started again. I believe in you, but you don't need to take my word for it. All you need is to trust that you can ask the right questions and take control where you need to.

Out of all the messages there are in this book, here is the one I want you to leave with. Ask questions and take control. I've said this so many times, but that's because it is so important that you do it. You won't know all of the answers if you aren't willing to ask the questions. We are all too comfortable with other people controlling our lives, but we shouldn't be. We must take responsibility. It is the only way we can ensure that we get everything that we need out of life. This is the one thing I want you to take away from this book.

It's a big scary world out there filled with so many lies. All I can hope is that I've helped you see the truth and have led you down the right path. Soon you'll be just like me, enlightened, healthy, and living a full and free life. Let's show those big industries that they don't own us and we aren't going to let them control us anymore. Now our duty is clear: to spread the knowledge we have. Don't let your friends and family suffer like we have. Spread the truth and snuff the lies until the world is free from the greedy businessmen and we are all able to live our best lives.

References

11 Foods to Increase Your HDL. (2019). *Healthline*. Retrieved 6 November 2019, from https://www.healthline.com/health/high-cholesterol/foods-to-increase-hdl#see-your-healthcare-provider

12 Little Weight-Loss Tricks Only Nutritionists Know. (2019). *The Healthy*. Retrieved 2 November 2019, from https://www.thehealthy.com/weight-loss/weight-loss-tricks-from-nutritionists/

13 Foods That Could Lower Your Risk of Cancer. (2019). *Healthline*. Retrieved 7 November 2019, from https://www.healthline.com/nutrition/cancer-fighting-foods#section6

America. Retrieved 7 November 2019, from https://thebreastcancercharities.org/10-cancer-causing-foods/ *Antibiotics*. (2019). Retrieved 8 November 2019, from https://www.hopkinsmedicine.org/health/wellness-and-prevention/antibiotics

Antibiotic Resistance: The Top 10 List. (2019). *Drugs.com*. Retrieved 8 November 2019, from https://www.drugs.com/article/antibiotic-resistance.html

Cancer, B., Cancer, C., Cancer, L., Cancer, P., Types, V., & Medicine, P. et al. (2019). *What foods and drinks are linked to cancer?. Cancer Treatment Centers of America*. Retrieved 7 November 2019, from https://www.cancercenter.com/community/blog/2017/10/what-foods-and-drinks-are-linked-to-cancer

Cancer Prevention Diet - HelpGuide.org. (2019). HelpGuide.org. Retrieved 7 November 2019, from https://www.helpguide.org/articles/diets/cancer-prevention-diet.htm

Eat Less Red Meat, Scientists Said. Now Some Believe That Was Bad Advice.. (2019). Nytimes.com. Retrieved 7 November 2019, from https://www.nytimes.com/2019/09/30/health/red-meat-heart-cancer.html

end-point measurement. (2019). TheFreeDictionary.com. Retrieved 2 November 2019, from https://medical-dictionary.thefreedictionary.com/end-point+measurement

Eric Metcalf, M., & Krystal Cascetta, M. (2018). *Photo Gallery: 10 Top Foods to Fight Cancer. EverydayHealth.com.* Retrieved 7 November 2019, from https://www.everydayhealth.com/cancer-photos/top-foods-to-fight-cancer.aspx

-->, <., -->, <., -->, <., -->, <., & -->, <. *(2019). Everything We Have Been Told Is A Lie - The Medical Industry Is Designed For Profit Not People! — Steemit. Steemit.com.* Retrieved 2 November 2019, from https://steemit.com/conspiracy/@jockey/everything-we-have-been-told-is-a-lie-the-medical-industry-is-designed-for-profit-not-people

Glucose Not Carbohydrates Fuel Our Brains | HealthCentral. (2018). Healthcentral.com. Retrieved 7 November 2019, from https://www.healthcentral.com/article/the-carbohydrate-brain-fuel-myth

guide, L., Book, U., Recipes, 2., Treats, 2., family, L., & boxes, L. et al. (2013). *The Food Pyramid - how they are wrong and why were they invented?. Ditch The Carbs.* Retrieved 2

November 2019, from
https://www.ditchthecarbs.com/why/food-pyramids/

guide, L., Book, U., Recipes, 2., Treats, 2., family, L., & boxes, L. et al. (2014). *Why high fat? Why low carb? Read all you need to know.. Ditch The Carbs.* Retrieved 2 November 2019, from https://www.ditchthecarbs.com/why/why-high-fat/

HDL (Good), LDL (Bad) Cholesterol and Triglycerides. (2019). *www.heart.org.* Retrieved 6 November 2019, from https://www.heart.org/en/health-topics/cholesterol/hdl-good-ldl-bad-cholesterol-and-triglycerides

HuffPost is now a part of Verizon Media. (2019). *Huffpost.com.* Retrieved 2 November 2019, from https://www.huffpost.com/entry/dont-trust-your-doctor_b_18977

Johnson, E., Johnson, E., Contributor, i., Garcia, A., Johnson, E., & Contributor, i. (2014). *The 10 Most Cancer Causing Foods - Breast Cancer Charities of America. iGoPink | Breast Cancer Charities of*

Khambatta, C. (2014). *Are Carbs Helping or Destroying Your Brain? | Nutrition and Fitness for Diabetes and Insulin Resistance. Nutrition and Fitness for Diabetes and Insulin Resistance.* Retrieved 7 November 2019, from https://www.mangomannutrition.com/carbs-helping-hurting-brain/

LaRosa, J. (2019). *Top 9 Things to Know About the Weight Loss Industry. Blog.marketresearch.com.* Retrieved 2 November 2019, from https://blog.marketresearch.com/u.s.-weight-loss-industry-grows-to-72-billion

MDLinx International. (2019). *Mdlinx.com.* Retrieved 2 November 2019, from https://www.mdlinx.com/internal-medicine/article/4008

Publishing, H. (2019). *11 foods that lower cholesterol - Harvard Health. Harvard Health.* Retrieved 6 November 2019, from https://www.health.harvard.edu/heart-health/11-foods-that-lower-cholesterol

Red meat, processed meat and cancer | Cancer Council NSW. (2019). *Cancer Council NSW.* Retrieved 7 November 2019, from https://www.cancercouncil.com.au/1in3cancers/lifestyle-choices-and-cancer/red-meat-processed-meat-and-cancer/

Should You Trust Your Doctor?. (2019). *Psychology Today.* Retrieved 2 November 2019, from https://www.psychologytoday.com/intl/blog/fighting-fear/201306/should-you-trust-your-doctor

The 3 Lies of Fitness. (2016). *Whole Life Challenge.* Retrieved 6 November 2019, from https://www.wholelifechallenge.com/the-3-lies-of-fitness/

Top 10 fitness lies - busted!. (2019). *Expertrain.com.* Retrieved 6 November 2019, from https://www.expertrain.com/blog/fitness/top-10-fitness-lies-busted.htm

The Corruption of Evidence Based Medicine — Killing for Profit. (2018). *Medium.* Retrieved 2 November 2019, from https://medium.com/@drjasonfung/the-corruption-of-evidence-based-medicine-killing-for-profit-41f2812b8704

This Is the Worst Diet Advice Nutritionists Have Ever Heard. (2019). *The Healthy.* Retrieved 2 November 2019, from https://www.thehealthy.com/nutrition/worst-diet-advice/

What Cholesterol Means for Your Heart. (2019). *WebMD.* Retrieved 6 November 2019, from https://www.webmd.com/cholesterol-management/features/cholesterol-bigger-picture#2

*Viral Infections - Why Don't Antibiotics Kill Viruses? -
Drugs.com*. (2019). *Drugs.com*. Retrieved 8 November 2019,
from https://www.drugs.com/article/antibiotics-and-
viruses.html

Made in the USA
Coppell, TX
23 February 2021

50723607R00069